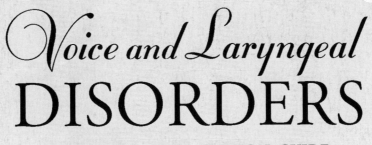

Voice and Laryngeal
DISORDERS

A PROBLEM-BASED CLINICAL GUIDE
WITH VOICE SAMPLES

W9-BXO-784

Voice and Laryngeal
DISORDERS

A PROBLEM-BASED CLINICAL GUIDE
WITH VOICE SAMPLES

TOURO COLLEGE LIBRARY
Kings Highway
WITHDRAWN

SALLY K. GALLENA, M.S., CCC-SLP

Graduate Instructor and Clinical Supervisor,
Department of Speech-Language Pathology & Audiology,
Loyola College in Maryland, Baltimore, MD

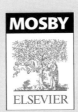

MOSBY

ELSEVIER

MW

MOSBY
ELSEVIER

11830 Westline Industrial Drive
St. Louis, Missouri 63146

Voice and Laryngeal Disorders
A Problem-Based Clinical Guide With Voice Samples

ISBN-13: 978-0-323-04622-0
ISBN-10: 0-323-04622-3

Copyright © 2007 by Mosby, Inc., an affiliate of Elsevier Inc.

All rights reserved. No part of this publication may be reproduced or transmitted in any form or by any means, electronic or mechanical, including photocopying, recording, or any information storage and retrieval system, without permission in writing from the publisher.
Permission is hereby granted to reproduce the *ASHA Code of Ethics* in this publication in complete pages, with the copyright notice, for instructional use and not for resale. Although for mechanical reasons all pages of this publication are perforated, only those pages imprinted with a Mosby, Inc., an affiliate of Elsevier Inc. copyright notice are intended for removal.

Notice

Neither the Publisher nor the [Editors/Authors] assume any responsibility for any loss or injury and/or damage to persons or property arising out of or related to any use of the material contained in this book. It is the responsibility of the treating practitioner, relying on independent expertise and knowledge of the patient, to determine the best treatment and method of application for the patient.

The Publisher

ISBN-13: 978-0-323-04622-0
ISBN-10: 0-323-04622-3

Publishing Director: Linda Duncan
Editor: Kathryn Falk
Developmental Editor: Andrew Grow
Project Manager: Tracey Schriefer
Design Direction: Teresa McBryan

Working together to grow
libraries in developing countries

www.elsevier.com | www.bookaid.org | www.sabre.org

ELSEVIER   BOOK AID International   Sabre Foundation

Printed in the United States of America

Last digit is the print number: 9 8 7 6 5 4 3 2 1

5/26/09

This book is lovingly dedicated to
my husband Rich;
my family, whose names appear in the case studies;
and to my "helper" who was ever-present throughout this project.

Sally

This book has evolved over several years while I have been teaching graduate level speech-language pathology students in voice disorder classes and supervising them in the clinic, and working with clients with voice and laryngeal disorders. The first part of the book is composed of case studies and accompanying audio voice samples of actual clients that the author has evaluated and treated. This format attempts to familiarize new clinicians with the broad spectrum of voice disorders, the pertinent information that a basic diagnostic protocol yields, and the process of interpreting diagnostic information that is foundational to making appropriate recommendations and determining a treatment plan. Although the 24 case studies represent only a small portion of the voice and laryngeal disorders that the voice care team may see, they are representative of what the clinician working in a school, clinic, or medical facility might encounter. The accompanying CD has audio samples of each client's voice recorded during the diagnostic evaluation and in some cases following treatment. The audio portion was prompted by listening to a group of master voice researchers: when asked what one piece of equipment was imperative in their voice lab, they unanimously replied, "The ear!" Developing a trained ear and accurately describing and rating what one hears is essential for the clinician treating voice disorders.

Part II of the book focuses on assessment, providing tools for the evaluation of voice and laryngeal disorders. It is a compilation of resources for perceptual, acoustic, and physiological assessments. Many of the resources have been created by the author and piloted by students and practicing speech-language pathologists. Other resources have been contributed by professionals in the speech-language pathology field and by colleagues in allied professions. Diagrams are included, as are sample reports written by other specialists of the voice care team, to further aid the student studying voice and laryngeal disorders.

Part III is the treatment section of the book. The information contained in that portion assists the speech-language pathologist in planning voice therapy, writing goals, tracking client progress, and reporting results. This information functions as a helpful supplement to a more comprehensive textbook on voice therapy techniques.

Parts IV and V, containing labs and "unsolved" case studies, are the result of the American Speech-Language-Hearing Association's new Knowledge and Skills Acquisition (KASA)[1] initiative for graduate student training. The goal of the KASA initiative is for clinical competencies to be learned through the acquisition and integration of knowledge and skills in nine communication areas. Voice, resonance, and respiration disorders are one of the nine areas. These disorders historically encompass a small part of the clinical caseload and thus provide students few opportunities for hands-on experience with such disorders. In response to this challenge, this book uses a problem-based learning approach through which students can complete four clinical labs (respiration, resonance, voice analysis, and alaryngeal speech); they require a minimum of materials, while still targeting specific ASHA knowledge and skills standards. In the course evaluations received by the author over the past 2 years that this approach has been used, students have commented on the practicality of the labs and the knowledge that was gained through this learning format.

The ten "unsolved" case studies in Part V are divided equally between adult and pediatric cases. The culminating experience for students using this book is being able to read each incomplete case study, listen to the voice sample, and then—using

---

1. American Speech-Language-Hearing Association: *New certification standards*, 2006. Retrieved February 28, 2006, from http://www.asha.org/about/membership-certification/new_standards.htm

the resources provided within the book and the knowledge gained through study—complete each case study. This involves choosing appropriate trial therapy techniques, summarizing the findings, providing appropriate recommendations, and creating a treatment plan that can be as general or specific as desired. The author has used the unsolved case studies previously for class projects; they have resulted in stimulating class discussions, demonstrations of therapy techniques, sharing of commercial and clinician-made materials, and an overall improvement in clinical thinking and writing proficiency.

Feedback from current graduate speech-language pathology students and new practicing clinicians, who have helped pilot this book, has been extremely positive. Its uses range from helping them prepare for the Praxis examination[2] to being a valuable clinical resource that provides examples and practical tools for diagnosis and treatment of voice and laryngeal disorders.

2. American Speech-Language-Hearing Association: *Praxis exam for speech-language pathologist*, Retrieved February 28, 2006, from www.asha.org/students/praxis/overview.htm

The author would like to express sincere gratitude to my supportive family, to Robin Samlan, M.S., M.B.A., CCC, speech-language pathologist in the Department of Otolaryngology Head & Neck Surgery at Johns Hopkins Medicine, my encouraging colleagues, the clients and students who have taught me much more than I've taught them, and two special angels—Leslie Terrell and Dorothy Flint.

CONTENTS

PART II

EVALUATION

PART III

TREATMENT

PART IV

LEARNING OPPORTUNITIES

PART V

"UNSOLVED" CASE STUDIES

Answers to Labs and Unsolved Case Studies (See CD for Answers)

CD-ROM CONTENTS
Evaluation Materials

Adult Case History
Child Case History
Voice Evaluation
Stroboscopy Evaluation Rating Form (SERF)
University of Wisconsin Videostroboscopic Ratings
Current Voice Research—ASHA Division 3—CAPE-V
Voice Rating Scale
Rainbow Passage
Towne-Heuer Passage
Voice Handicap Index
Reflux Symptom Index
Speech and Voice Tasks for Assessing Spasmodic Dysphonia
Speech and Voice Tasks for Assessing Resonance
Male-to-Female Transgender Communication Assessment Form
Vocal Cord Dysfunction Patient Interview
Habit Cough Patient Interview

Therapy Materials

Voice Therapy Progress Note
Treatment for Vocal Cord Dysfunction
Treatment for Habit Cough
Cough Management Chart
Voice Care Tips
Laryngopharyngeal Reflux Information
Sources of Caffeine

Learning Opportunities (with Answers)

Respiration Lab
Voice Analysis Lab
Resonation Lab
Alaryngeal Speech Lab

UNSOLVED CASE STUDIES (WITH ANSWERS)

CASE STUDIES

You are about to read 24 case studies of clients that have received evaluations by a speech-language pathologist (SLP). Twenty-three have been clients evaluated by the author. The case study of Joseph, illustrating tracheoesophageal voice and speech was contributed by Robin Samlan, M.S., M.B.A., CCC, speech-language pathologist in the Department of Otolaryngology Head & Neck Surgery at Johns Hopkins Medicine. The accompanying CD will allow you to hear the client's voice. Prior to each case study, an overview of the disorder is provided to familiarize the reader with the general diagnostic and treatment information relevant to the disorder. The reader will note that the term *client* is used more often in this book than *patient*. "Client" denotes someone using the services of a speech-language pathologist or other professionals, whereas "patient" denotes being under the medical care of a professional.[51] Within our college clinic, we see individuals with a variety of disorders and differences, making the label *client* seem more appropriate than *patient*.

Most of the case studies follow a similar format, with the exception of the laryngeal disorders, such as vocal cord dysfunction, in which voice may not be problematic. The reason the person has come for the evaluation and his or her pertinent medical, voice, and social history information is discussed first. The importance of taking a thorough case history and listening with one antennae to what is being said, another to the sound of the voice, and a third to what is *not* being said, cannot be emphasized strongly enough. Likewise, asking open-ended questions, and not suggesting answers the clinician wants to hear, will assist the client in being comfortable and forthright in sharing information.

Often visual, auditory, and behavioral observations are included, especially when they provided additional input regarding the diagnosis or treatment. Being observant and able to describe what one hears and sees without being judgmental or jumping to conclusions is a sign of a mature, perceptive clinician.

The evaluation follows. Telling clients what is expected of them and demonstrating the tasks for them will aid their learning and increase their comfort level. For each voice disordered client, voice is subdivided and evaluated according to pitch, quality, loudness, respiration, and voice abuse behaviors. An integrated approach of perceptual and acoustic measures is provided for each case. Additional areas of the evaluation that may be included are the Voice Handicap Index score,[36] and comments about resonation, articulation, and oral motor skills (included especially when the client presents with a profile that could be consistent with a neurological disorder). When describing and rating the voice, the author has tried to consistently use the terminology that is part of the Consensus Auditory Perceptual Evaluation of Voice (CAPE-V),[8] in conjunction with a 5-point equal interval rating scale, where 1 denotes mild and 5 denotes severe. Each case study voice sample was described and independently rated by the author and Robin Samlan, M.S., M.B.A., CCC-SLP. Interrater agreement for each case was extremely high, differing maximally by 1 point on the 5-point scale.

Descriptions of the findings from laryngeal imaging information are provided for each voice case. Minimally each client presenting with a voice disorder was examined with a flexible or rigid laryngoscope. Stroboscopy findings, when available, also are included.

Copyright © 2007 by Mosby, Inc., an affiliate of Elsevier Inc. All rights reserved.

After the evaluation, trial therapy recommendations are given. Techniques that may improve voice or yield additional diagnostic information regarding the voice or laryngeal disorder are tried. The appropriateness of the chosen techniques is based on what is known about the vocal fold structure and function, the etiology, and the client. The results of trial therapy, if positive, can be extremely motivating to the client and can provide valuable prognostic information to the clinician.

The summary attempts to capture the most salient aspects of the evaluation in several paragraphs.[32] Busy recipients of reports may have time to read only the summary and recommendations; thus it is important that although brief, the summary is also as informative as possible. Recommendations are provided following the summary or included separately as a bulleted list. They vary depending on the client and the disorder, but typically encompass those points of action that the clinician feels are important, whether or not direct therapy is recommended and received.

Finally, each report contains a long-term goal as well as short-term goals. Goal writing is confusing to students and practicing clinicians alike—varying from institution to institution.[45] For this book, goals are regarded as those that would yield a successful treatment outcome if met. Thus long-term goals are treatment outcome goals—those that are realistic and hopeful given the client, his or her voice or laryngeal disorder, and potential obstacles encountered in the treatment process. Short-term goals represent the "road map" or delineation that will be followed to achieve the long-term treatment outcome goal. From these short-term goals, treatment session goals and plans are formulated. My colleagues and graduate students have illustrated that multiple clinical paths can be followed when treating voice disorders and that no single "recipe" is *the* path for a successful treatment outcome; it must simply be appropriate for the disorder and the client.

For some case studies, additional information is provided to let the reader know "the rest of the story." It is important that the student be exposed to the successes and failures that occur within our clinical caseload and recognize the limitations within our profession, as well as the value of other professional disciplines, as we collaborate in the care of the client.

Copyright © 2007 by Mosby, Inc., an affiliate of Elsevier Inc. All rights reserved.

The case study of Lydia is included in this book for several reasons: the pathology, the surgical technique and its impact on the layer structure of the vocal folds, the lack of speech pathology services before and immediately after surgery, and the age of the client. Thus, from Lydia, the speech-language pathologist can learn much.

Lydia had bilateral Reinke's edema, also known as *polypoid degeneration*. It is an accumulation of fluid in Reinke's space (the superficial layer of the lamina propria), usually covering the membranous portion of both vocal folds. In some cases, it is so diffuse and floppy that it interferes with respiration. Reinke's edema, although it does sometimes occur in adult males, is seen most often in adult females who have had a long history of cigarette use. A lowered habitual pitch is most characteristic of Reinke's edema, due to the added mass causing the vocal folds to vibrate more slowly. Additionally, because of the effect of extra mass on the vocal folds, increased subglottal pressure is required to allow vocal fold vibration. Thus the typical client will complain of a lower-pitched voice and strain and effort accompanying speaking.

Treatment options depend on the severity of the edema and the client's needs, ranging from voice therapy to surgery. Lydia had vocal fold stripping,[15,17] a surgical procedure that ablates the pathology without attempting to preserve the mucosa of the vocal fold edge. It is least desirable for voice preservation because of the potential for scar tissue development that negatively impacts vocal fold vibration. Lydia did not feel that she had been adequately counseled about the impact of the surgery on her voice. Her initial thought upon hearing her voice postoperatively was that "something big had gone wrong." Referral to a speech-language pathologist who is knowledgeable about voice disorders, both before the surgery and immediately, after, would have greatly benefited this client both vocally and psychologically.

Finally, Lydia represents the geriatric population that typically is unfamiliar with the profession of speech-language pathology and even less familiar with the subspecialty of voice with its abstract therapy techniques. Making the therapy concrete, functional, and relevant to Lydia's life was a stimulating challenge for the clinician.

Copyright © 2007 by Mosby, Inc., an affiliate of Elsevier Inc. All rights reserved.

CASE STUDY 1-1

Postoperative Reinke's Edema

Voice clip #1

BACKGROUND AND REASONS FOR REFERRAL

Lydia, a 79-year-old female, was seen for a voice evaluation at this clinic upon referral from her otolaryngologist. The presenting complaints were ongoing vocal strain, hoarseness, and voice loss after surgery for Reinke's edema. Her daughter, who assisted in providing pertinent information, accompanied Lydia.

HISTORY

According to Lydia, 2 months of worsening hoarseness, voice breaks, low pitch, and inability to talk loudly prompted Lydia's initial consultation with an otolaryngologist. She was diagnosed with Reinke's edema (polypoid degeneration) and underwent surgical vocal fold stripping of both folds for removal of the edema approximately 1 month before this evaluation. Lydia had not been referred to a speech-language pathologist before the surgery. After surgery, the client observed 2 days of complete voice rest. Aphonia and severe hoarseness were reported by the client when she resumed speaking. According to client report, she was not provided with postoperative instructions for voice use other than to observe 2 days of voice rest. Though gradual voice improvement has been noted, both Lydia and her daughter feel that her present voice quality is worse than it was before surgery. Voice is reportedly strongest in the morning and worsens with continued voice use. A repeated laryngoscopic examination performed 1 week before this evaluation revealed progress in vocal cord healing, with residual swelling of both vocal folds. Voice therapy was recommended by the otolaryngologist.

Before this surgery, history was positive for cigarette use, approximately one pack per day for 45 years. She has now stopped smoking. Caffeine intake is estimated at four beverages daily. Noncaffeinated fluid intake is good. Lydia takes Norvasc and Toprol for hypertension. She does not drink alcohol. No symptoms of laryngopharyngeal reflux (LPR) are experienced. No known allergies are reported, though periodically she has sinus drainage.

Lydia has worked outside of her home since she was a teen. Most of her jobs have required excessive talking over competing background noise. Presently, Lydia is married and does not work outside her home. She reported a long history of marital distress, which has been further affected by her voice problems in conjunction with her husband's hearing loss, negatively impacting their ability to communicate with one another. She describes feelings of depression, unexplained sadness, and lethargy.

EVALUATION
Pitch

Fundamental frequency pitch range was 114-380 Hz, approximately 14 whole notes, which is below normal limits. Habitual pitch (speaking fundamental frequency [SFF]) was estimated at 131 Hz, but fluctuated. Perceptually, using a 5-point ascending severity rating scale, pitch rating was a 3, corresponding to a moderate deviancy. SFF is not within normal limits for her age and gender. Frequency perturbation was 5.41, which greatly exceeds normal limits and correlates perceptually with the dysphonic voice.

Quality

On a 5-point severity rating, roughness and strain were rated as 4 (moderate to severe), whereas breathiness was rated as 2 (mild to moderate). Phonation breaks and hard glottal attacks occurred frequently. Overall voice severity was rated as 4 (moderate to severe).

Copyright © 2007 by Mosby, Inc., an affiliate of Elsevier Inc. All rights reserved.

Loudness

Appropriate for the treatment room with no background noise. Loudness decayed with continued talking. Attempts to increase loudness significantly increased vocal strain.

Respiration

Normal abdominothoracic breathing patterns were observed. Maximum phonation duration (MPD) for /a/ averaged 12 seconds, which is within normal limits for her age and gender. S:Z ratio was 1.5 (20 and 13 seconds, respectively), which is not within normal limits and suggests increased airflow through the glottis during phonation.

Vocal Abuse Behaviors

The following vocal abuses were reported as excessive by the client:
> Shouting and yelling
> Talking over noise
> Excessive talking
> Coughing and throat clearing

Voice Handicap Index

The Voice Handicap Index (VHI) scale, which seeks to assess the level of impact caused by the voice problem within three areas: physical, emotional, and functional, was rated by the client on a 0 to 4 severity scale (0 = never; 4 = always).
Total VHI score: 76/120
> *Subscale scores:*
> 27/40 Physical
> 24/40 Functional
> 25/40 Emotional

Resonation

Within normal limits.

Articulation

Within normal limits without dysarthria.

TRIAL THERAPY

At the conclusion of this evaluation, the client was counseled on the negative effects of voice misuse and phonotrauma on vocal fold healing. Additionally, she was acquainted with the "sound" and "feel" of strained, effortful phonation. Directives to speak easier, yet not whisper, were given, which resulted in reduced effort. She was instructed in humming frequently throughout the day in an easy voice, feeling for vibration in her nose and mouth.

SUMMARY

This 79-year-old female presents with postsurgical roughness, strain, and breathiness after bilateral vocal fold stripping for polypoid degeneration 1 month before this voice evaluation. Despite good intentions, the client has continued to use her voice excessively and effortfully, often in her communication with her husband. She has stopped smoking after 45 years of cigarette use. She expresses depression and frustration associated with her voice and its impact on day-to-day communication.

Trial voice therapy targeting reduced effort and resonant focus produced a slight improvement in overall voice quality. Voice facilitative techniques were abstract to Lydia, thus humming was chosen as a means to reduce effort. Lydia's daughter appeared to have a good understanding of what was taught and agreed to assist her mother with practice.

Copyright © 2007 by Mosby, Inc., an affiliate of Elsevier Inc. All rights reserved.

RECOMMENDATIONS

1. 6 sessions of trial voice therapy with continued treatment based on the progress achieved and the client's satisfaction with her voice.
2. Discussion of the case with the referring otolaryngologist. Request copies of all pertinent information.
3. Laryngeal videostroboscopy to assess and document vocal fold structure and function and for client education purposes.
4. Marriage counseling, with a recommendation for a hearing evaluation for Lydia's husband with an audiologist.

Long-term Goal

- Lydia's voice will be acceptable to her and audible and understandable to others at a conversational loudness level, as reported by the client and her family.

Short-term Goals

1. The client will reduce vocal abuse and misuse by 50% as assessed through charting and client report.
2. The client will make modifications in her home environment to promote better communication with her spouse.
3. The client will improve hydration by substituting two noncaffeinated drinks for two caffeinated ones.
4. The client will observe a minimum of three 30-minute vocal rest periods daily.
5. The client will use voice facilitative techniques (humming, chanting, etc.) to reduce vocal effort, as assessed through perceptual and acoustic documentation.

Copyright © 2007 by Mosby, Inc., an affiliate of Elsevier Inc. All rights reserved.

Three very different case studies are presented here to illustrate vocal cord dysfunction (VCD), also referred to as *paradoxical vocal fold motion (PVFM)*.[47] The first is Elise, a 14-year-old athlete, whereas the second is Nan, a 37-year-old nurse. The third is Regina, a 61-year-old administrator.

VCD is a condition in which the vocal folds move in a paradoxical manner during the breath cycle, adducting on inhalation or, in some cases, adducting on both inhalation and exhalation (biphasic), causing dyspnea and apnea.[16] The tightness is localized to the larynx with associated stridor. It often accompanies aerobic exercise, being experienced by the athlete when at maximum physical demand. It is frequently misdiagnosed as exercise-induced asthma (EIA), but does not respond to typical asthma treatment. VCD is being reported with increased incidence in the medical profession.

Several conditions are hypothesized to contribute to or cause VCD, most notably laryngopharyngeal reflux (LPR),[61] also termed *gastroesophageal reflux disease (GERD)*; allergies; and sinusitis, with the latter two causing chronic postnasal drip. Morrison and Rammage (1999)[46] have proposed the term *irritable larynx syndrome (ILS)*, which encompasses muscle tension dysphonia, chronic cough, globus, and VCD. They hypothesized that these conditions are triggered by physical or emotional factors causing a neurologically mediated "spasm-ready" response by the larynx and vocal folds. While Nan experienced only dyspnea (thus there is no voice recording for her), Elise had dysphonia and VCD symptoms. Regina's chief complaint was a persistant cough, though dysphonia and VCD were present to a lesser degree.

This author's experience is that VCD is most often diagnosed by a pulmonologist through pulmonary function testing, as well as additional testing (exercise or chemical) to intentionally trigger a VCD episode. Laryngeal imaging with stroboscopy is an important tool for ruling out LPR and chronic postnasal drip and for assessing vocal fold movement, whether asymptomatic or symptomatic.

Therapy by a speech-language pathologist is the treatment of choice, in conjunction with medication as needed if an underlying medical condition exists. Psychotherapy is sometimes recommended to address stress management and performance anxiety, the latter for athletes.

This author has had extensive experience treating clients with VCD, (predominantly athletes). A VCD evaluation form is included in the diagnostic section of this book; therapy techniques are included in the treatment section.

Copyright © 2007 by Mosby, Inc., an affiliate of Elsevier Inc. All rights reserved.

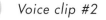

CASE STUDY 2-1

Vocal Cord Dysfunction

Voice clip #2

BACKGROUND AND REASONS FOR REFERRAL

Elise, a 14-year-old ninth grade female, was referred to this clinic for an evaluation and therapy. She complains of breathing difficulty accompanying strenuous dancing. She was diagnosed with VCD by a pediatric pulmonologist after extensive testing. Elise's mother accompanied her to this appointment, which included office and exercise components.

HISTORY

Elise has experienced breathing problems while dancing during the past 6 months that have increased in frequency and severity. She reported that the first episode occurred when performing a dance solo. Following that, she was seen by her pediatrician, who suspected that she had exercise-induced asthma. She began using an inhaler before exercise, but noted no improvement in symptoms. After repeated pediatrician appointments, Elise was referred to a pulmonologist for a clinical examination, which included pulmonary function tests with flow-volume studies, a methacholine challenge to rule out asthma, and a treadmill stress test to produce VCD symptoms. A laryngoscopic examination was not done. All tests supported a diagnosis of VCD. A referral for speech pathology services was made.

Presently, she notes that after 1 to 2 minutes of dancing she has difficulty inhaling and begins gasping for air. She rated the severity of symptoms as moderate to severe, experiencing throat tightness, stridor, and occasional dizziness. She describes the onset of symptoms as sudden, accompanying her need for more air. Resting temporarily stops the symptoms; however, they recur with exercise onset. She has not required emergency assistance.

Elise participates on her school dance team, performing hip-hop–style dance, in addition to dance lessons for jazz, tap, and ballet. She dances 4 to 5 times a week for a total of approximately 13 hours.

Elise is in good health. History is negative for asthma. She denies reflux symptoms. She has been taking Zyrtec as needed for allergies. No other medications are taken. History is negative for neurological abnormalities. She is currently receiving counseling for "social issues." She describes herself as independent, smart, outgoing, and a perfectionist. She is the younger of two siblings and lives with her mother and father.

OBSERVATIONS

Elise presented as a thoughtful, intelligent teenager. She seemed very interested in knowing more about VCD and willingly participated in all therapy activities.

Elise demonstrated a fast-paced 2-minute hip hop routine that would typically trigger VCD symptoms. Her breathing during this was characterized by frequent shallow inhalations, without a consistent rate or rhythm. Intermittently breath holding was observed. A high level of upper body tension was observed in response to the upper torso involvement of the dance. She appeared to be in excellent physical condition.

EVALUATION
Pitch

Within normal limits for age and gender.

Quality

Mild to moderate roughness and strain (2 on a 5-point severity rating). Glottal fry and occasional hard glottal attacks noted.

Copyright © 2007 by Mosby, Inc., an affiliate of Elsevier Inc. All rights reserved.

Loudness

Within normal limits.

Musculoskeletal Tension

Palpation of the larynx revealed a reduced thyrohyoid space with increased laryngeal elevation.

Respiration

Expiratory reserve volume was used consistently, as she spoke with lengthy breath groups.

Overall Severity

Mild; she stated that her voice had sounded like this as long as she could remember, and it did not interfere with her communication.

LARYNGOSCOPIC FINDINGS

Erythema of the posterior larynx and the glottal surface of the epiglottis area suggestive of LPR was seen. One slight abnormal respiratory movement of the folds was noted after a glissando where the arytenoids were noted to quickly adduct before the respiratory abduction. No other incidences of paradoxical motion were seen. During phonatory tasks a muscle tension pattern with significant anteroposterior supraglottic constriction was noted, which is consistent with her voice quality.

TREATMENT

Therapy focused on:
1. Developing an understanding of normal vocal fold movement during respiration.
2. Developing an understanding of VCD as well as its possible triggers.
3. Learning breathing training techniques to be used to reduce VCD symptoms:
   a. Sensing signs of VCD, staying calm, focusing on exhalation rather than inhalation.
   b. Prolonging exhalation while hissing or blowing through pursed lips.
   c. Using a short, gentle, well-supported inhalation from the diaphragm.
   d. Using a consistent breathing rate and ratio of greater exhalation time to inhalation time.
4. Using positive visual imagery and self-talk.
5. Transferring the breathing technique to stretching exercises as well as dance.
6. Planning ways to implement breathing training techniques into dance routines.

SUMMARY

This 14-year-old highly motivated female athlete presents with VCD while dancing. Additionally, her voice evidences roughness and glottal fry consistent with muscle tension dysphonia. Laryngoscopic findings were consistent with LPR and muscle tension dysphonia. A breathing technique was taught that focused on using supported abdominal inhalation and lengthened exhalation; establishing a breathing rate that is rhythmic with the counts and steps of the dance routine. Elise demonstrated an understanding of the above concepts but found it very challenging to implement them while dancing. This was addressed by having her slow her breathing rate while dancing by breathing equal intervals on counts of four. Though inhalation and exhalation cycles were of equal duration, she provided feedback that this "felt better." While stretching, she was able to implement VCD breathing as instructed.

RECOMMENDATIONS

1. Discuss laryngeal findings with her physician for diagnosis and reflux management.
2. Maintain a consistent rhythmic breathing rate when learning new dance routines so that the breathing technique can be maintained when the dance is brought up to normal speed.

Copyright © 2007 by Mosby, Inc., an affiliate of Elsevier Inc. All rights reserved.

3. Find less strenuous "rest periods" within the dance when VCD breathing can be used.

4. Refrain from breath holding while dancing.

5. At the conclusion of the dance, continue to use VCD breathing until respiration rate returns to normal and feelings of throat tightness subside.

6. Practice VCD breathing for several brief periods per day, during inactive periods as well as during exercise to develop comfort with it.

7. Participate in ongoing therapy at this clinic to address VCD and muscle tension dysphonia, because the latter may be contributing to an overall tense laryngeal posture.

Long-term Goal

■ Elise will dance for two successive hip hop dances (approximately 7 minutes) without symptoms of VCD interfering with her performance as assessed through client report.

Short-term Goals

1. To establish and maintain VCD breathing during stretching, dancing, and cooling down.

2. To learn voice and laryngeal facilitative techniques that will reduce laryngeal muscle tension and promote voice quality that is within normal limits.

Copyright © 2007 by Mosby, Inc., an affiliate of Elsevier Inc. All rights reserved.

CASE STUDY 2-2
Vocal Cord Dysfunction

BACKGROUND AND REASONS FOR REFERRAL

Nan, a 37-year-old wife, mother, and practical nurse, was referred for a speech pathology evaluation secondary to a diagnosis of VCD by her allergist.

HISTORY

Nan stated that she has had symptoms consistent with VCD intermittently for the past 11 years. Presumed to be asthma, it has been treated with asthma medications. During a recent hospitalization due to breathing difficulty, she was examined by an otolaryngologist, who observed paradoxical vocal fold movement characteristic of VCD. The otolaryngologist's examination revealed signs of reflux, for which Prevacid was prescribed. Nan was then referred to an allergist for allergy and asthma assessments. The allergist's testing was consistent with mild asthma in addition to VCD. It was then recommended that Nan consult with a speech pathologist and a psychologist or psychiatrist.

Symptoms described are throat and upper chest tightness followed by stridorous, labored breathing. She notes no consistency regarding possible triggers for the episodes; however, she questions allergies, fumes, fragrances, and stress. Though she states that she does not panic in response to an episode, when they occur at work, it is insisted that she go to the emergency room for evaluation and treatment. She stated that she hoped today's speech pathology appointment would allow her to learn control strategies for the VCD symptoms so that she can continue her work.

Nan describes her overall health as good. She had a cervical fusion for chronic degenerative disc disease 2 years ago without complications. She has allergies that are treated with immunotherapy. Noncaffeinated fluid intake is good. She does not smoke. Benadryl is taken nightly to aid sleep. She has been taking Paxil for the past year, prescribed by her family physician. This was triggered by her awareness of an abnormal level of anxiety when her son began driving a car. She denies conflict associated with family or work relationships.

OBSERVATIONS

Nan was very pleasant throughout the evaluation. She seemed genuinely motivated to get maximum benefit from the information imparted and the techniques taught. Her breathing throughout the interview was comfortable without signs or symptoms of tension or anxiety. Her voice did not evidence roughness or strain.

TREATMENT

VCD was explained and illustrated through use of a model of the larynx and a videotape showing the paradoxical movement of the vocal folds during a VCD episode. The video illustrated how a forceful inhalation "deep breath" intensifies the paradoxical adductor action of the vocal folds. Likewise, it illustrated that sniffing improved vocal fold abduction, as did gentle transnasal inhalation.

A breathing technique was then taught focusing on a short, but supported, abdominothoracic inhalation through the nose, followed by a lengthened exhalation, sustaining /s/ (i.e., hissing) with the breath out. A comfortable rhythm and ratio of inhalation to exhalation was established. Nan was reminded to maintain the feeling of an "open throat" and to keep her upper torso relaxed. Additionally, visual imagery and relaxing music were used to create a calm atmosphere. Through role-playing and practice Nan seemed to have a good understanding of the behavioral and cognitive skills that were taught.

Copyright © 2007 by Mosby, Inc., an affiliate of Elsevier Inc. All rights reserved.

SUMMARY

This 37-year-old female presents with VCD of many years duration. It appears that there are many triggers for VCD—asthma, reflux, chronic postnasal drip, chemical odors, and anxiety. Patient education and instruction on VCD and breathing techniques were the focus of today's session. Nan was instructed regarding the need to practice the breathing technique frequently so that it can become a learned response to the sensations that signal VCD. Progress will be monitored through weekly charting of practices and symptoms and through phone conversations, with additional sessions scheduled as needed.

RECOMMENDATIONS

1. To focus on the exhalation phase of the breathing cycle, phonating a hissing sound while lengthening exhalation.
2. To use a breathing rhythm and ratio where exhalation exceeds inhalation.
3. To reduce upper body tension in response to VCD.
4. To resist the urge to take "deep inhalations" when experiencing VCD; rather to sniff or inhale gently through the nose.
5. To use positive mental imagery and calm self-talk when experiencing symptoms to reduce associated anxiety.

Long-term Goal

▪ Nan will have increased control over her VCD, by effectively using breathing retraining strategies, as assessed by posttreatment ratings of severity and frequency of attacks.

Short-term Goals

1. Nan will demonstrate accurate VCD breathing, using a consistent breathing rhythm and ratio and diaphragmatic breathing, in the therapy room for 3-minute intervals, five times during the session.
2. Nan will use positive mental imagery and instructional self-talk when role-playing VCD attacks.
3. Nan will teach VCD respiratory retraining techniques to her husband and a coworker so that they can guide her in their use during a VCD episode.

Copyright © 2007 by Mosby, Inc., an affiliate of Elsevier Inc. All rights reserved.

CASE STUDY 2-3

Irritable Larynx Syndrome

BACKGROUND AND REASONS FOR REFERRAL

Regina, a 61-year-old female, presents with irritable larynx syndrome (ILS), manifested in a habitual cough and paradoxical vocal fold motion of several years duration. She was referred by her otolaryngologist and was accompanied by her husband to this evaluation.

HISTORY

According to Regina, upper respiratory infections have typically triggered a habitual cough pattern. More recently, she noticed that strong odors associated with chemicals, smoke, and paint also trigger coughing. She was previously diagnosed with asthma and treated pharmacologically for many years. Since being recently evaluated at a specialty medical center by a pulmonologist and otolaryngologist, asthma and allergies have been ruled out. Regina has been reluctant in accepting this based on her symptoms, which include a sensation of "fluid" in her lungs and airway. She has been diagnosed with LPR and is taking medication and making lifestyle and diet adjustments.

The client describes herself as frustrated and weary due to cough frequency and severity. She stated that it interferes with her social, work, and home life. She describes her job as one of high pressure and feels that stress exacerbates the cough problem. She describes herself as upbeat, and talkative but prone to stress. She currently takes Singulair and Flonase, as well as Pepcid and Zoloft, the latter medication as needed. She expressed a feeling of hopelessness regarding a cure for her cough.

LARYNGEAL EXAMINATION

Upon laryngeal examination using a flexible nasolaryngoscope, slight paradoxical vocal cord motion was observed at rest when the patient had no awareness of symptoms. When asked to take a deep breath, the vocal folds moved medially, with lateral-medial and anterior-posterior compression observed. The vocal folds were observed to abduct normally when the patient was instructed to exhale. Through guided transnasal "sniffing" followed by purposeful exhalation, vocal fold movement was normalized, although with each deep inhalation attempt they initially moved in an adducted direction prior to abducting. Coughing was not observed during this examination.

OBSERVATIONS

Regina initially presented as very disheartened and anxious about her cough. At times she was tearful when talking about her situation, describing it as "frustrating and weary." She questioned what benefit could be achieved from a "speech therapist." She became more comfortable as the session continued. Although she wasn't feeling well, she participated in all activities. Regina coughed for an extended period every 5 to 10 minutes, with several episodes requiring her to expectorate saliva or mucous. She described an intense sensation prior to coughing that cannot be ignored. No symptoms of VCD such as stridor or difficulty inhaling (apart from coughing) were noted.

EVALUATION
Laryngopharyngeal Reflux

The Reflux Symptom Index (RSI), which assesses LPR symptoms during the past month using a 0 (no problem) to 5 (severe problem) rating scale, was rated by the client. Her score was 29/45 possible points; the authors consider a score above 12 to be suggestive of LPR. Rated as 4s and 5s were excess throat mucous; difficulty swallowing foods, liquids, pills; and troublesome or annoying cough.

Copyright © 2007 by Mosby, Inc., an affiliate of Elsevier Inc. All rights reserved.

Voice

Pitch, loudness, and quality were within normal limits for age and gender. Mild strain and roughness (rated as 1 on a 5-point scale) were noted.

Respiration

Normal breathing patterns noted when not coughing. No stridor or dyspnea observed. Frequent sighing noted during the interview.

TREATMENT

Regina was educated and instructed in alternatives to coughing, with each technique practiced during the session. Techniques taught included the following:
1. Blowing through the urge or the actual cough with tightly pursed lips.
2. Swallowing slowly and deliberately (liquid or saliva) in response to the cough urge as in "massaging" the larynx with the swallow.
3. Learning and practicing gentle diaphragmatic inhalations in a supine or comfortable seated position, to counteract her rapid, effortful upper chest inhalations that occur before coughing.
4. Learning laryngeal massage. This was taught to both the client and her husband.

She made an effort to use the techniques when coughing, which she stated possibly delayed the cough response. She would, however, eventually cough with ferocity. She felt that relaxed diaphragmatic breathing and laryngeal massage were most beneficial in reducing and controlling the cough.

SUMMARY

Regina presents with symptoms consistent with ILS, triggered, it appears, by respiratory infections, chemicals and fumes, and stress. She evidences symptoms of anxiety and depression, though it is not known whether her emotions trigger ILS or are the outcome of ILS. At the time of the evaluation, there were no clinical signs of VCD, thus the cough was targeted. Cough management strategies were introduced and practiced. She continued to cough during the practice, but expressed positive feelings toward laryngeal massage and diaphragmatic breathing.

The diagnosis, symptoms, and proposed treatment were discussed with the client and her husband. Regina was assured that the symptoms are genuine and are amenable to treatment provided by a speech-language pathologist familiar with the diagnosis. It is felt that she will need multiple sessions to effectively treat the cough.

It was also suggested that Regina seek counseling for stress management. Several names of counselors in her geographical area were given to her.

RECOMMENDATIONS

1. Participate in speech therapy to learn cough reduction techniques and desensitization techniques for odor tolerance.
2. Participate in counseling for stress and anxiety management.
3. Continue to make diet and behavioral modifications in addition to taking medicine for reflux control.

Long-term Goal

- Regina will use cough reduction strategies to reduce the frequency and severity of her cough episodes, thereby allowing her to attend work and social functions, as reported by the client and her husband.

Short-term Goals

1. Regina will comply with LPR management strategies, as monitored through client report and a decreased score on the Reflux Symptom Index.
2. Regina will use cough reduction strategies as needed to reduce the frequency and severity of cough episodes as evidenced through ongoing charting.

Copyright © 2007 by Mosby, Inc., an affiliate of Elsevier Inc. All rights reserved.

Clients with a diagnosis of habit cough, sometimes called *chronic psychogenic*, or *tic cough*, are being referred with increasing frequency to the speech-language pathologist for therapy. The profile of the client varies depending on whether he or she is a child or an adult. A typical child with habit cough initially developed the symptom as a result of an upper respiratory infection, where the cough lingered long after the infection cleared. Often such children report feeling a "tickle" or "bubble" in their throat that necessitates coughing. The cough varies in sound (ranging from a bizarre honking sound to a normal cough sound), frequency of occurrence (multiple times per minute to several coughs per day); and severity (interfering with school attendance). Diagnosis is made based on a normal physical exam (usually with radiographic studies), unresponsiveness to medication, and an absence of cough while sleeping.

Certain factors may cause or exacerbate habit cough; thus it is important that these be considered. They are (1) laryngopharyngeal reflux (LPR), (2) chronic postnasal drip, (3) neurological disorders such as Tourette's syndrome, and (4) psychological problems whereby the person unconsciously is seeking attention and receiving gain through coughing.

Adults with habit cough (or habit throat clear) typically have had a long-standing history with the problem and are less convinced that the problem is habit based verses organically caused. Ruling out (or medically treating) LPR, as well as any condition that may cause airway hypersensitivity, is extremely important, as is a thorough investigation of all medications taken and possible side effects. Because of the strength of the habit and the ferocity of the cough (some patients routinely cough until they gag or vomit), as a whole treating adults is often more challenging in regard to achieving a successful treatment outcome. Refer to Regina's Case Study 2–3.

Treatment of habit cough combines behavioral and cognitive therapy approaches. This author has found that teaching the client to respond to the "tickle" with a response that is incompatible with coughing, such as blowing or whistling, in conjunction with gentle, relaxed inhalation, is very effective. In an unpublished treatment outcome study by this author presented at the 2006 ASHA Convention of 14 male and 14 female children with habit cough (mean age 11 years), therapy provided by an SLP was successful for 82% of the children, with 71% of the parents rating the therapy as "very effective."[26]

An evaluation form for habit cough is included in the diagnostic section of this book. Treatment goals and a chart for documenting the use of cough reduction techniques are found in the treatment section of this book.

Copyright © 2007 by Mosby, Inc., an affiliate of Elsevier Inc. All rights reserved.

CASE STUDY 3-1

Habit Cough

BACKGROUND AND REASONS FOR REFERRAL

Alex, a 10-year-old male, presented with excessive cough of 4 weeks duration after a referral from his allergist. Alex's mother accompanied him to this evaluation.

HISTORY

Alex's problem started with a cold approximately 4 weeks before this evaluation; the viral infection resulted in excessive coughing. His prior medical history includes allergies and asthma, for which he is medicated with Advair, Singulair, Clarinex, and Rhinocort. History is also positive for LPR, for which he takes Prevacid. In response to the cold and persistent cough, he was prescribed cough medicines. Most recently Clonidine has been tried to reduce cough frequency. None of the medications have significantly improved the frequency of the cough.

An ENT evaluation revealed edema and erythema of the vocal folds, without evidence of lesion formation. The posterior glottis evidenced erythema, suggestive of reflux. Normal vocal fold movement was observed during voice production. Taking a deep breath immediately triggered a cough.

When interviewed about his cough, Alex indicated that it was very bothersome to him, made him tired, and at times made his head hurt. He stated that he feels a constant "tickle" in his throat requiring him to cough. He has missed the past five school days due to the disruptive nature of the cough. Questions regarding stress or worry did not reveal an obvious psychogenic component. With regard to cough pattern and frequency, he indicated that it was consistent across activities and time of day. However, the cough is absent at night. There is no evidence of neurological problems, and no family history of Tourette's syndrome.

Alex is the youngest of three children. His mom described him as friendly, outgoing, compassionate, and eager to learn. Additionally, she noted that he frustrates easily, is sensitive, and dramatic. Mother denies abnormal stress or conflict in the home. Alex has never participated in counseling services.

OBSERVATIONS

Alex willingly participated in all treatment activities. He was attentive and mature acting for his age. No tic type behaviors were visually observed by the clinician.

EVALUATION
Voice

Mild roughness, presumably resulting from the vocally abusive nature of the cough was noted; pitch and loudness perceptually were within normal limits.

Respiration

Intermittent, irregular inhalation presumably caused by attempts to stifle coughing was observed. Breathing was most rhythmic and regular when Alex was speaking.

COUGH OBSERVATIONS

Two types of coughs were heard: (1) a normal sounding cough that occurred at the frequency of one cough per 15 seconds and (2) one that resembled a sneeze, heard with less frequency. Intermittently a hard throat clear was also heard. The longest interval between coughs occured when Alex was conversing.

TREATMENT

The cause and effect of habitual coughing was explained to Alex. The cyclical nature of habit cough was compared to a mosquito bite where repeated scratching increases

Copyright © 2007 by Mosby, Inc., an affiliate of Elsevier Inc. All rights reserved.

sensitivity and strengthens the habit. He was instructed in alternatives to coughing and guided in their use. Techniques taught included the following:

1. Swallow hard (liquid or saliva) or slowly in response to the "tickle" or urge to cough.
2. Substitute blowing through pursed lips or making a hissing sound before coughing when the urge is perceived or after the initial cough to break the cough sequence.
3. Adopt "gentle," slow, abdominal breathing followed by a longer exhalation with blowing or hissing during periods of coughing; refrain from taking a deep breath.
4. Substitute an effortful /h/ sound for the cough or throat clear.
5. "Turn the voice on." That is, sing, count, speak to keep the vocal folds engaged.

Alex rehearsed these techniques repeatedly, showing understanding of the techniques. During 10 separate trials in which the goal was to use a cough reduction technique in place of coughing or to interrupt the cough sequence, his ability to control his cough varied from 30 seconds to 5 minutes. It took great effort and concentration, as well as clinician cueing for this success because his desire to cough was intense.

SUMMARY

This 10-year-old male presents with habit cough of approximately 4 weeks duration following an upper respiratory infection. The frequency with which he was coughing at the time of this evaluation was remarkable. Habit cough was explained and treatment techniques were taught. Upon completion of the session, he verbalized and demonstrated multiple ways that he could reduce or control the cough. He experienced initial success with cough control during this session, which suggests a positive treatment outcome. Information on various food and environmental triggers for cough, as well as a list of treatment techniques, and a chart to tally practice success were given to the client and his mother.

RECOMMENDATIONS

1. Review cough reduction strategies throughout the day, tallying their success for minimally three 10-minute periods per day.
2. Focus on wellness and give the cough less attention.
3. Encourage conversation with Alex to determine whether he has bothersome psychosocial issues.
4. Provide information to the school nurse, teacher, and guidance counselor to increase their knowledge of habit cough.
5. Return to this clinic for weekly or twice weekly therapy sessions.
6. Schedule for laryngeal imaging to examine structure and function of the vocal folds.

Long-term Goal

■ Alex will break the habit of coughing in all situations, as reported by the client, his parents, and his teacher.

Short-term Goals

1. Alex will reduce the frequency of his cough by 75% through the use of cough reduction strategies, with performance charted for minimally three 10-minute periods per day.
2. Alex will be able to consistently attend school, without trips to the nurse's office, through the use of behavioral and cognitive cough control strategies.

Copyright © 2007 by Mosby, Inc., an affiliate of Elsevier Inc. All rights reserved.

MUSCLE TENSION DYSPHONIA

This category of voice and laryngeal disorders seems most confusing to students studying voice disorders, at least in part, because of its multiple labels, descriptions, and etiologies. Historically, voice problems where there were no structural changes to the vocal folds were called "functional," whereas those with changes to the vocal fold mucosa were called "organic." Those categories, however, become "muddied" when pathologies such as vocal nodules and polyps are discussed. The same etiologies (voice misuse and overuse), causing similar negative perceptual voice characteristics (hoarseness, breathiness, and strain), might not cause vocal fold pathology in one person, while causing nodules or a polyp in another person. All the while, the underlying muscle pattern is the same, one of hyperfunction (i.e., too much effort). Whether a pathology develops from muscle hyperfunction or just a voice deviancy without pathology, the speech-language pathologist's role is the same: to treat the functioning of the laryngeal system.

In this book the term *muscle tension dysphonia (MTD)*, first used by Morrison, Nichol, and Rammage[47] will be used to describe those voice disorders resulting from laryngeal muscle hyperfunction without structural change to the vocal folds. In an attempt to help the reader cross reference terminology, additional labels will be provided as well. For example, Sarah and Sean both appeared to have a psychogenic trigger for the onset of MTD. Thus the characteristics of this type of voice disorder will be presented before their case studies. MTD with mucosal change such as vocal nodules, polyps, and cysts will be presented separately.

Copyright © 2007 by Mosby, Inc., an affiliate of Elsevier Inc. All rights reserved.

MUSCLE TENSION DYSPHONIA WITHOUT MUCOSAL CHANGE

This group of muscle misuse voice disorders is as varied as the labels under which it is classified. Its onset can be sudden (as when cheering at a sporting event) or gradual (developing over the course of months or years). It can occur following an upper respiratory infection or as part of one's unique personality. It can affect pitch, loudness, and quality or only a single component of voice. It can result in aphonia when the tense folds are abducted or dysphonia when they are adducted. It can be disabling to the speaker or merely a nuisance. It can be further aggravated by medical conditions or develop as a compensatory response to another underlying problem.

Despite the variety of presentations inherent in the label "muscle tension dysphonia," there appears to be one overriding consistency: The speaker is incorrectly using muscles for voice production, causing changes in the acoustic signal and sensory complaints.

Common causes of MTD are overuse (i.e., abuse) and misuse of the larynx and vocal folds. Various medications, chronic medical conditions (i.e., reflux), and ongoing exposure to irritants contribute to the problem, as do changes in emotional and physical health.

Certain professions[64] (those of teachers, clergy, singers, and professional voice users) and avocations (sport participants and enthusiasts) seem to have an increased risk for developing MTD because of high voice demands.

As stated previously, the voice and laryngeal effects of MTD vary in range and severity. This is observed perceptually, acoustically, and aerodynamically. The most common voice characteristics are roughness, breathiness, and strain, with accompanying pitch and phonation breaks, and hard glottal attacks. Phonation range may be reduced or show evidence of a break. Speaking quietly is often more challenging than talking at elevated loudness levels. Complaints of vocal fatigue, throat irritation and dryness, and an increased desire to clear the throat are frequent. Likewise, visible and palpable signs and symptoms of excessive musculoskeletal tension in the upper torso and larynx are present.

Laryngostroboscopic findings show a wide range of abnormality with regard to vocal fold closure patterns, ventricular and supraglottal lateral compression, anteroposterior compression, vocal fold amplitude, mucosal wave, phase closure, symmetry, and periodicity of successive vibratory cycles.[18] Most commonly one would expect to see a wide posterior gap (chink) upon closure, medial and anteroposterior compression of the glottis and supraglottis, reduced vocal fold amplitude, a lengthened closed phase, and vibratory aperiodicity.[61]

Voice therapy is effective in reducing or eliminating MTD. Length of treatment varies widely, with gradual onset, long-standing MTD usually requiring more therapy than sudden-onset aphonia or dysphonia. Reducing laryngeal hyperfunction can be accomplished through a variety of treatment approaches used most often in combination: symptomatic (Confidential Voice,[17] yawn-sigh, chanting,[15] etc.); etiological (reducing vocal abuse, improving vocal hygiene); tension reduction (laryngeal massage[11] and relaxation); and physiological (Resonant Voice Therapy[72] and Vocal Function Exercises[69]).

Copyright © 2007 by Mosby, Inc., an affiliate of Elsevier Inc. All rights reserved.

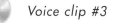

CASE STUDY 4-1

Muscle Tension Dysphonia

Voice clip #3

BACKGROUND AND REASONS FOR REFERRAL

Justin, an 8-year, 8-month-old male third grader, was seen for a voice consultation upon referral from his speech-language pathologist. Justin experiences chronic vocal hoarseness and intermittent aphonia. The referring speech-language pathologist has seen him for an evaluation and three voice treatment sessions. She questions the effectiveness of her treatment because of a lack of progress with regard to Justin's voice quality. Justin was accompanied by his mother, who served as the informant.

HISTORY

Justin's voice has been hoarse for as long as his mother can recall. She has observed an increase in the amount of effort that Justin uses to produce voice. She feels that his voice quality is fairly consistent with regard to time of day and year. According to mom, Justin does not seem overly concerned by his voice problem, but complains that his throat sometimes feels dry and tired, and occasionally it is hard for him to get his "voice out."

An otolaryngologist, who performed flexible nasoendoscopy prior to the referral for voice therapy, reported fullness on the medial margin of both vocal folds at the anterior one-third, posterior two-thirds juncture. Additionally, anteroposterior squeezing was observed accompanying phonation.

Justin is the fourth of seven children. No other siblings are reported to have voice problems. Justin is very active with outside play and sports. He also loves to sing. Regarding school and sports performance, Justin's mother stated that he puts a great deal of pressure on himself to excel. Despite many children in the home, an excessively noisy home environment was denied.

Justin's birth and developmental history were described as medically unremarkable. His mother did not recall him crying excessively as a baby, nor having an abnormal sounding cry. He did not have colic. He had one episode of croup associated with flu symptoms at age 4 years that required short-term hospitalization. He has had no surgeries or injuries to the head or neck.

Currently Justin is in good health. History is negative for allergies, postnasal drip, enlarged tonsils or adenoids, and gastroesophageal reflux. He takes no medications on a regular basis. His fluid intake is good. He sleeps well.

Justin's voice therapy goals have focused on reducing effort, decreasing vocal abuses, and improving vocal hygiene.

EVALUATION
Pitch

Speaking fundamental frequency (SFF) was estimated at 275 Hz, which is within normal limits for his age and sex. Very few pitch inflections were heard during conversation. Phonation range (when asked to sing a scale), was 262-466 Hz, approximately eleven semitones, which is not within normal limits. When trying to imitate a siren, difficulty was experienced maintaining phonation, due to multiple aphonic breaks.

Quality

Overall severity was rated as 4 on a 5-point scale (moderate to severe). Breathiness and strain were rated as 4 (moderate to severe), whereas roughness was rated as a 2 (mild to moderate). Many aphonic breaks were heard, ranging in duration from a syllable to several successive words. During 1 minute of reading, 10 aphonic breaks were noted from a total of 103 words (10%). Likewise, during a 1-minute prompted monologue

Copyright © 2007 by Mosby, Inc., an affiliate of Elsevier Inc. All rights reserved.

of 50 words, eight aphonic breaks were heard (16%). There appeared to be no phonemic pattern; however, more breaks occurred toward the ends of breath groups. Hard glottal attacks were also present.

Loudness

Appropriate for a small group setting. He was noted to have difficulty maintaining consistent conversational loudness levels for a prolonged period without becoming aphonic. Voice quality was less hoarse when speaking at elevated loudness levels.

Respiration

Normal breathing patterns were observed during rest. Breathing for speech, however, appeared shallow and was focused in the upper chest. Maximum phonation duration (MPD) for /a/ averaged 14 seconds, which is within normal limits for his age. Four phonation breaks accompanied sustained phonation. S:Z ratio was 0.94 (16 and 17 seconds, respectively), which indicates no significant discrepancy between phonation and respiration.

Musculoskeletal Tension

Excessive prominence of laryngeal strap muscles, particularly the sternocleidomastoids, was observed when phonating. Laryngeal structures, when palpated, seemed unremarkable. Laryngeal massage produced a marginal change in voice quality.

Vocal Abuse Behaviors

The following factors were identified as possible contributors to Justin's dysphonic voice:

 Yelling, and loud talking associated with sports and play
 Use of an effortful whisper
 Overall amount of singing
 Overall amount of talking

Resonation

Within normal limits.

Articulation

Within normal limits.

Language

Age appropriate.

TRIAL THERAPY

Justin was educated on the auditory and visual signs of excessive vocal effort observed when he talked, specifically effortful phonation, aphonic voice breaks, and the visual appearance of excessive muscle tension in his neck. He was shown exercises to relax his neck, throat, and shoulders. He was guided in the use of supported breathing, while yawning and phonating sustained vowel sounds ("yawn-sigh" facilitative technique). There was a noticeable improvement in his voice using this technique, which was tape recorded for future sessions.

SUMMARY

This 8-year-old male presented with a voice that is characterized by hoarseness, strain, multiple aphonic phonation breaks, and reduced pitch range. Dysphonia has been ongoing since early childhood. The results of a laryngeal examination suggested MTD that is maintained by a pattern of voice abuse and overuse (which cause hoarseness and breathiness), followed by a compensatory response of increased intrinsic and extrinsic laryngeal muscle tension (his method to achieve a better voice).

Copyright © 2007 by Mosby, Inc., an affiliate of Elsevier Inc. All rights reserved.

RECOMMENDATIONS

1. Videostroboscopy to assess laryngeal structure and function and to rule out a vocal fold cyst.
2. Continued voice therapy for six additional sessions, assessing progress through acoustic, perceptual, and observational methods.
3. Modify those vocal behaviors and personality characteristics that trigger inappropriate amounts of tension and abusive voice use.
4. Consult a trained singing instructor for singing evaluation and instruction.
5. Parental involvement in the therapy process for increased carryover of treatment goals.

Long-term Goal

- Justin will acquire and maintain less effortful voice production in normal noise settings that is without voice breaks as reported by the client and his parents.

Short-term Goals

1. Justin will reduce vocal abuses in all settings by 50%, as determined through charting and family report.
2. Justin will reduce MTD through the use of voice facilitative techniques as assessed through the CAPE-V with an overall severity level of 2 or less.
3. Justin will increase hydration by drinking an additional 24 oz of noncaffeinated fluids daily.

Copyright © 2007 by Mosby, Inc., an affiliate of Elsevier Inc. All rights reserved.

MUSCLE TENSION DYSPHONIA SECONDARY TO LARYNGOPHARYNGEAL REFLUX (LPR)

The speech-language pathologist treating swallowing and voice disorders has become increasingly more familiar with the symptoms, signs, and treatment for reflux. The original diagnosis of gastroesophageal reflux disease (GERD) included digastric as well as laryngopharyngeal complaints. In the *Classification Manual for Voice Disorders I*[73] GERD and LPR have been classified as distinctly different disorders, based on the presence or absence of laryngeal involvement.

Reflux refers to the backflow of gastric contents from the stomach into the esophagus and hypopharynx. It is experienced to some degree by everyone, most often following meals. When there is evidence of laryngeal inflammation and irritation with concomitant voice complaints such as roughness, breathiness, soreness, vocal fatigue, habit coughing, and chronic throat clearing, it becomes problematic. Over time, the irritation causes mucosal changes leading to chronic laryngitis, contact ulcers, and contact granulomas.[43] It also is associated with increased tone in the muscles of the larynx and pharynx, contributing to MTD.[61]

Upon laryngoscopic examination for LPR, the larynx and vocal folds will be seen as reddened and swollen. The posterior glottis is generally more affected than the anterior glottis because of the proximity of the esophagus to the arytenoids and cartilaginous portion of the vocal folds. If a space-occupying lesion has developed as a result of the chronic irritation, the vibratory characteristics of the vocal folds will reflect the structural changes.[61]

Often the speaker has no obvious symptoms of reflux such as heartburn, and if not probed for other symptoms or examined carefully, the diagnosis may go undetected. The evaluation form included in the diagnostic section of the book will guide the SLP in probing for symptoms. Included as well is the Reflux Symptom Index,[12] a scale that allows clients to review and rate their reflux symptoms over the course of a month, yielding a total score that serves as both a diagnostic and posttreatment tool.

Treatment for LPR typically involves pharmacological intervention with diet and lifestyle modifications, often combined with voice therapy. Medications (of which the most popular group is proton pump inhibitors) used to manage reflux are described in the "Guide to Vocology" from the National Center for Voice and Speech.[71] Treatment suggestions are provided on their website as well (www.ncvs.org/). An additional information sheet on reflux management is included in the treatment section of this book. Appropriate voice therapy techniques are those used to reduce MTD that have previously been discussed.

Copyright © 2007 by Mosby, Inc., an affiliate of Elsevier Inc. All rights reserved.

CASE STUDY 4-2

Muscle Tension Dysphonia Secondary to Laryngopharyngeal Reflux (LPR)

Voice clip #4

BACKGROUND AND REASONS FOR REFERRAL

Judith, a 53-year-old professional, was seen for a voice evaluation. She complains of hoarseness, intermittent pitch breaks, and frequent coughing. Flexible nasoendoscopy revealed a diagnosis of LPR.

HISTORY

Judith first noticed hoarseness and voice loss approximately 2 months before this evaluation. She described the onset as sudden. Since that time, her voice has gradually improved but has not returned to "normal." At the time of this evaluation, Judith described her voice as hoarse, with frequent pitch breaks. She stated that she cannot project her voice or sing as she had been able to do in the past. She also reported the feeling of food "sticking" in her throat and a feeling of "fullness" (globus) in her throat. She reported that the voice problem impacts both her professional life and her personal life.

Using the Reflux Symptom Index (RSI), Judith scored reflux symptoms over the course of the past month as 34 out of 45 possible points. (The authors of the RSI suggest that a score greater than 12 is significant for reflux.) She indicated a severe problem (ratings of 5) with hoarseness; presence of an annoying cough (most frequent after eating or when lying down); and the sensation of something sticking in her throat. A score of 4 was given to throat clearing and difficulty swallowing food, liquids, or pills. Since starting on Prevacid, 3 weeks before this evaluation, she feels that her symptoms have improved somewhat.

Judith reports having allergies and asthma, which are controlled by medication as needed. She also reports having an anxiety disorder with occasional panic attacks. She is currently taking the following medications regularly: Prevacid, Dexedrine, Diovan, and Effexor. Fluid intake is excellent with minimal caffeine use. She does not smoke or drink alcohol. She reports her home and work environments as dusty.

Judith lives with her husband. She works long hours during the week and spends weekends volunteering with several organizations.

LARYNGEAL EXAMINATION

Edema and erythema of the arytenoid cartilages and cartilaginous portion of the vocal folds with tissue hypertrophy of the posterior glottis. No evidence of contact ulcer(s) or granuloma(s) was found. Stroboscopy revealed medial compression of the vocal folds with a large posterior glottal chink. Mucosal wave was reduced with thick mucous stranding across the vocal folds.

EVALUATION
Pitch

Fundamental frequency for sustained /a/ was 205 Hz. Speaking fundamental frequency in contextual speech was 174 Hz, which is low for her age and gender. Fundamental frequency pitch range was 133-348 Hz, approximately 11 whole tones, which is not within normal limits. Frequency perturbation for /a/ was 2.85, correlating perceptually to vocal hoarseness.

Copyright © 2007 by Mosby, Inc., an affiliate of Elsevier Inc. All rights reserved.

Quality

Breathiness was rated as 4 (moderate to severe), roughness as 2 (mild to moderate), and strain as 3 (moderate). Phonation breaks and hard glottal attack phonation initiation were heard. Voice quality was consistent throughout the evaluation.

Loudness

Appropriate for a conversational setting. Mean loudness was 77 dB.

Vocal Abuse Behaviors

The following abuses were identified and rated on a 0 to 5 scale (5 most frequently occurring).

    5—Coughing
    4—Talking excessively; throat clearing
    3—Singing

Respiration

Abdominothoracic breathing patterns were observed. Maximum phonation duration for sustained /a/ was 9 seconds, which is not within normal limits for age and gender.

Resonation

Within normal limits.

TRIAL THERAPY

Resonant Voice Therapy techniques were introduced to Judith. Her resultant voice evidenced reduced strain and an elevated pitch level.

SUMMARY

This 53-year-old female presents with vocal strain, breathiness, roughness, phonation breaks, and a low-pitched voice suggestive of MTD caused by LPR. She feels that her voice has improved since starting medication and instituting diet changes, although it is still deviant, which negatively impacts her communication effectiveness. It is felt that she would benefit from voice therapy to reduce her hyperfunctional manner of phonation, improve and maintain reflux management, and substitute less abusive vocal behaviors for those in which she is currently engaging. Prognosis for improved voice is favorable based on client's self-disciplined personality and the improvement that has been experienced thus far through medical intervention.

RECOMMENDATIONS

1. Voice therapy for 4-6 sessions.
2. Follow behavioral guidelines for reflux management.

Long-term Goal

■ Judith will establish and maintain a voice that is within normal limits perceptually, allowing her to resume regular voice demands at home and at work, as assessed by the CAPE-V and client report.

Short-term Goals

1. Judith will reduce vocal hyperfunction through use of voice facilitative techniques, specifically Vocal Function Exercises performed twice daily.
2. Judith will increase speaking fundamental frequency by three semitones, thereby using a pitch level that is more efficient for her vocal folds.
3. Judith will decrease and monitor LPR through regular use of behavioral modification and medication, minimally reducing her score on RSI by 10 points.

Copyright © 2007 by Mosby, Inc., an affiliate of Elsevier Inc. All rights reserved.

MUSCLE TENSION DYSPHONIA OF PSYCHOLOGIC ORIGIN: PSYCHOGENIC VOICE DISORDERS

It has long been recognized that a person's emotional state is reflected in his or her voice. Normal responses to emotions are evident in one's habitual pitch and pitch inflections, overall loudness, voice quality, nonverbal vocalizations, and speech rate. This variation is normal when temporary and occasional. However, when voice abnormality is ongoing, or extremely deviant, without a physical cause, often there is a psychological cause.[11] Although many classifications of mental and behavioral disorders have abnormal voice, speech, and language components, voice evaluation and therapy is used most often for stress-related and somatoform disorders.[43] Voice disorders within these categories seem to present with some distinct features that alert the speech-language pathologist to a possible psychogenic etiology. Some of these features are further defined in the literature as conversion voice disorders.

General features of psychogenic MTD are as follows:

- Normal vocal fold structure despite abnormal hyperfunction (adducted or abducted).
- Inconsistency in the severity of dysphonia or aphonia accompanying certain situations, persons, topics, and emotions.
- Vegetative voice functions (throat clear, cough, laugh) that sound normal.
- Elevated laryngeal position, reduced thyrohyoid space, and muscle pain associated with laryngeal palpation.
- Client reaction to the voice problem that does not accurately reflect the severity of the problem (exaggerated or understated).
- Onset of dysphonia may be sudden, not attributable to illness, trauma, or vocal abuse.
- A recent upper respiratory infection or bout of infectious laryngitis.
- Client description of a recent stressful event or ongoing anxiety and/or depression preceding the voice problem.
- Primary and secondary gains achieved through the voice disorder at an unconscious level.
- Responsiveness to behavioral voice therapy techniques that reduce musculoskeletal tension and cognitive techniques such as suggestion.
- Voice improvement that is often dramatic, occurring within a very short time (one session).

For clients with presumed psychogenic MTD, the speech-language pathologist's role is to assess and treat laryngeal function; observe, question, and acknowledge the client's psychological and emotional status (information on which is included in the diagnostic and treatment sections of the book); explain the links between the voice problem, emotional status, and muscle function; and recognize when a referral for a psychological consultation is appropriate and necessary.[11]

Copyright © 2007 by Mosby, Inc., an affiliate of Elsevier Inc. All rights reserved.

CASE STUDY 4-3

Muscle Tension Dysphonia of Psychological Origin

 Voice clip #5

BACKGROUND AND REASONS FOR REFERRAL

Sarah, a 41-year-old government employee, was seen for a voice evaluation upon referral from her otolaryngologist. She complains of sudden voice loss and severe hoarseness lasting for 14 days.

HISTORY

According to client report, voice loss occurred suddenly, which was attributed to an upper respiratory infection. However, when cold symptoms lessened, voice did not improve. Sarah was seen by her otolaryngologist for flexible nasoendoscopy 3 days before this voice evaluation. According to physician report, her vocal cords were normal in appearance with mild edema and erythema and reduced adduction of the true vocal folds when phonating.

Throughout this evaluation, she exhibited frequent throat clearing, with a strong sound. She complained of ongoing throat pain and tightness. Sarah denied having previous voice problems. She uses her voice extensively at work, but denies a history of voice abuse. No other family members have voice problems. She has no family history of neurological disease. She denies allergies. Occasional reflux symptoms are experienced and treated with antacids. History is negative for intubation, surgery, or trauma to the head or neck.

Because of the presumed psychogenic nature of this client's voice disorder, possible reasons for sudden voice loss were explored, specifically conflict and stress at home or in the workplace. Sarah disclosed that there was an ongoing conflict at work between a co-worker and herself, both of whom had recently vied for the same promotion. The co-worker had gotten the promotion, making the dynamics of the workplace very uncomfortable. Because of voice loss, Sarah had not been at work for the past week. Sarah participated in counseling for a few sessions at the outset of the work conflict.

EVALUATION (PRETREATMENT)
Pitch

Pitch was not measured for the aphonic voice. Speaking fundamental frequency for dysphonia during the reading of a passage ranged from 142-320 Hz.

Quality

Voice was predominantly aphonic, with severe strain. Quality was inconsistent, ranging from aphonia to severe dysphonia, with supraglottal phonation heard.

Loudness

Variable depending on voice quality.

Respiration

Shallow, effortful breathing was observed.

Musculoskeletal Tension

The larynx and strap muscles were sensitive to palpation. The larynx was elevated with a reduced thyrohyoid space.

Copyright © 2007 by Mosby, Inc., an affiliate of Elsevier Inc. All rights reserved.

Voice Handicap Index

The Voice Handicap Index (VHI) scale, which seeks to assess the level of impact caused by the voice problem within three areas: physical, emotional, and functional, was rated by the client on a 0 to 4 severity scale (0 = never; 4 = always).
Total VHI score: 65/120
Subscale scores:
27/40 Physical
21/40 Functional
17/40 Emotional

TRIAL THERAPY

It was explained to Sarah that she had "forgotten" how to naturally produce her voice and that her strong throat clear confirmed her ability to phonate. Using a throat clear to initiate voice, in conjunction with laryngeal massage, Sarah's voice was restored. Additional facilitative techniques such as humming, chanting, and use of upward pitch inflections were used to improve the naturalness of her voice.

It was further explained that often voice loss that is sudden, with no systemic illness, has a psychological cause, triggered by anxiety, stress, or interpersonal conflict. Additionally, the voice disorder sometimes functions to allow the person to physically or verbally avoid the difficult situation. Sarah identified with this information and agreed to resume counseling if the work situation did not improve.

EVALUATION (POSTTREATMENT)
Pitch

Pitch was stabilized at 175 Hz, which was low for her age and sex. Pitch inflections were implemented with increased voice use.

Quality

With voice treatment techniques, quality progressed from aphonia and severe dysphonia to phonation that was within normal limits. Initially very guarded in her attempts to phonate, voicing became more automatic and less effortful with increased use.

Loudness

Perceptually within normal limits for a small group setting. Mean intensity was 65 dB.

Respiration

Abdominothoracic breathing was reestablished. Sarah rested a hand on her abdomen as a reminder to use "full" (not deep) breaths.

Musculoskeletal Tension

Laryngeal position was lowered. Thyrohyoid space was increased and softened. Larynx and strap muscles remained sensitive to palpation, though reduced as compared to pretreatment.

SUMMARY

This 41-year-old female presented with a MTD of psychological origin of 2 weeks duration. Voice was restored during this session using voice facilitative techniques and laryngeal massage. Pretherapy and posttherapy acoustic and perceptual measures were taken. The nature of the voice disorder was discussed with the client, and reasons for the sudden voice loss were explored. She has agreed to continue psychological counseling if she feels that it is indicated. Additionally, the treatment sequence used to regain voice was written and reviewed for her, so that it could be self-implemented if necessary.

Copyright © 2007 by Mosby, Inc., an affiliate of Elsevier Inc. All rights reserved.

RECOMMENDATIONS

1. To continue using a conversational level voice in all settings, targeting smooth, automatic voice with normal pitch inflections.
2. To maintain good vocal hygiene.
3. To review the therapy sequence that was used to regain voice, if she experiences further voice problems.
4. To resume counseling to gain insight on conflict resolution and in how to improve communication in the work environment.

Long-term Goal

- Sarah will continue using a voice that is functional and within normal limits for her age and gender, in all communication situations, as reported by the client.

Copyright © 2007 by Mosby, Inc., an affiliate of Elsevier Inc. All rights reserved.

CASE STUDY 4-4

Muscle Tension Dysphonia of Psychological Origin

Voice clip #6

BACKGROUND AND REASONS FOR REFERRAL

Sean, a 20-year-old resident college student, was seen for a voice evaluation upon self-referral. He complained of intermittent voice loss and tongue weakness lasting for approximately 1 month.

HISTORY

According to client report, intermittent voice loss occurred over the course of 2 days approximately 1 month after entering college. He attributed it to having the flu. Initially he described his voice as "catching," where he had "trouble starting words." His voice continued to worsen, and he began having trouble moving his tongue to articulate words. He returned to his home town and was examined by an otolaryngologist, where he was told that he had laryngitis, prescribed antibiotics, and told to rest his voice. Voice did not improve following a course of antibiotics. He then went to the college health center, where he was sent to a reputable medical center for further evaluation. By this time his speech was difficult to understand; he was unable to participate in class discussions and was feeling very frustrated. His larynx was again examined through flexible nasoendoscopy, which resulted in insignificant findings and a diagnosis of laryngitis, despite a normal throat clear. Sean communicated with the physician by writing because he was unable to be understood. Speech therapy was recommended if voice did not improve in a week.

Sean has had no previous voice, speech, or language concerns. He denied symptoms of reflux and does not have allergies. He has had no surgeries or injuries to the head and neck. He takes no medications regularly. Fluid intake has been increased over the past month. Noncaffeinated fluid intake consists of two beverages per day. He denies excessive alcohol use and does not smoke cigarettes.

At the time of this evaluation, Sean was continuing to go to all of his classes but was unable to participate in class discussions, which he feared was impacting his grade in most classes. He was concerned about his health, indicating that he questioned whether there was a tumor that had not been discovered. Aside from his communication problem, he felt relatively well, though he was beginning to isolate himself from other students because of his frustration and the awkwardness of their questions and comments. When asked about life stress before the development of his voice problem, he disclosed that he was new to the college, having gone to a community college near his home. He professed that he was enjoying college, but that it was academically more challenging than his previous school.

Sean came to the college speech and hearing clinic hopeful that an improvement could be made in his voice and speech.

OBSERVATIONS

Sean was noticeably upset when he came for the evaluation. He communicated through writing, having written his concerns before coming to the evaluation. When encouraged to speak, it was noted that he rarely moved his tongue, which negatively affected articulation. Tongue movement was noted, however, when he swallowed. During the evaluation he cleared his throat, producing a sound that was much stronger than his attempts at voicing. He complained of throat pain, tightness, and dryness.

Copyright © 2007 by Mosby, Inc., an affiliate of Elsevier Inc. All rights reserved.

EVALUATION (PRETREATMENT)
Pitch

Due to voice fluctuation, pitch was not measured. Bursts of true voice were perceived as occurring at a pitch that is within normal limits for age and gender. Phonation range could not be measured.

Quality

Overall voice severity rating was 5 (severe). Aphonia and strain were rated as 5 (severe) with bursts of normal phonation occurring frequently but randomly.

Loudness

Soft for a small group setting because of aphonia.

Respiration

Shallow, effortful breathing was observed.

Musculoskeletal Tension

The larynx was elevated and the suprahyoid muscles were very sensitive to palpation.

Voice Handicap Index

The Voice Handicap Index (VHI) scale, which seeks to assess the level of impact caused by the voice problem within three areas: physical, emotional, and functional, was rated by the client on a 0 to 4 severity scale (0 = never; 4 = always).
Total VHI score: 82/120
  Subscale scores:
  25/40 Physical
  25/40 Functional
  32/40 Emotional

Articulation

When speaking, tongue posture was forward in the mouth with tongue tip tucked against the bottom incisors; reduced lip movement and closure were seen. Speech was unintelligible, with best articulation heard on vowel sounds.

TRIAL THERAPY

Cough, throat clear, laugh, and brief bursts of humming were performed volitionally with "true" voice. Tongue movement was generated by having the client chew with exaggerated tongue motion and having him observe his tongue in the mirror. Based on his performance with these skills, it was suggested to Sean that he had the potential for clearer voice. Using a throat clear to "turn on his voice," and lengthening the throat clear to produce a forceful hum, Sean began sustaining phonation for longer periods of time without allowing his voice to break. Jaw and laryngeal massage were used to reduce musculoskeletal tension. Voice could then be initiated with a hard glottal attack and sustained. Progression through sustained vowels with exaggerated articulator movement was next introduced, with automatic speech following. By the conclusion of the session, voice and articulation were within normal limits, yet very guarded and deliberate in execution. Pretherapy and posttherapy audio recordings were made for purposes of comparison.

SUMMARY

This 20-year-old male presented with MTD that affected articulation as well. Voice was restored during the evaluation session. Practice suggestions were given, as well as positive suggestion that his voice would continue to get stronger with increased use. The nature of the voice disorder was discussed with the client, and reasons for the sudden voice change were explored. The client did not feel that his communication

Copyright © 2007 by Mosby, Inc., an affiliate of Elsevier Inc. All rights reserved.

problem was linked to emotions associated with the changes to which he is adjusting. He has agreed to consult the college counseling center if further problems are experienced.

RECOMMENDATIONS

1. To continue using a conversational level voice in all settings, targeting smooth, automatic voice and articulation.
2. To maintain good vocal hygiene.
3. To review the therapy sequence that was used to regain normal voice and speech, if he experiences further voice problems.
4. To monitor emotional health, checking in with the college counseling center, if prolonged symptoms of depression or anxiety are experienced.
5. To call his family and share the news of his restored voice.
6. To direct professors to contact the evaluating SLP with any questions.
7. To send report copies to the ENTs that were consulted, to educate them on psychogenic MTD voice disorders.

Long-term Goal

■ Sean will continue using a voice that is within normal limits for his age and gender, in all communication situations, as reported by the client.

Copyright © 2007 by Mosby, Inc., an affiliate of Elsevier Inc. All rights reserved.

This voice disorder is known by varying names: *puberphonia, mutational falsetto, functional falsetto, adolescent transitional voice disorder* to name a few. These labels all describe the same phenomenon: an inappropriately high-pitched voice in an individual who is transitioning through (or has completed) puberty.[17] This is most commonly seen in males, often caused by rapid, dramatic voice change or unsettled, fluctuating voice change causing the speaker to want to maintain his higher "safer" pitch.

Laryngostroboscopic findings reveal tight closure of the cartilaginous portion of the vocal folds, with the membranous portion stretched tight and thin, so that vibration is confined to the medial edge of the vocal folds. Mucosal wave is reduced in accordance with reduced amplitude of vibration. In concert this produces a falsetto sound. Glottal closure pattern in conjunction with a lengthened open phase gives the voice a breathy quality.

Diagnostic indications for puberphonia are maintenance of a high-pitched voice that sounds mismatched to the speaker, pitch breaks (usually downward), lower-pitched throat clear, cough, and laugh. When observing the speaker, it is important to look for signs that puberty has occurred, such as facial and leg hair and larger thyroid cartilage with a more pronounced thyroid notch (Adam's apple).

Voice therapy using techniques such as laryngeal massage and manually lowering the larynx,[63] using vegetative functions[15] such as cough to establish appropriate pitch, and pushing and laryngeal isometrics[17] is effective for treating puberphonia. Helping the client comfortably transition into his "new" voice presents a challenge to both the patient and clinician.

Copyright © 2007 by Mosby, Inc., an affiliate of Elsevier Inc. All rights reserved.

NOTES

CASE STUDY 5-1

Puberphonia Voice Disorder

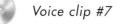 *Voice clip #7*

BACKGROUND AND REASONS FOR REFERRAL

Travis, a 15-year-old high school sophomore, was seen for a voice evaluation upon referral from his school SLP. Travis complained of "hoarseness," which has been present for the past year.

HISTORY

Travis did not identify pitch as the most deviant aspect of his voice; rather he described his voice as "hoarse." He noted that hoarseness is consistent throughout the day. He has learned to talk in a controlled manner whereby voice sounds better but restricts loudness. When asked about the pitch of his voice, he commented that he didn't think it sounded like his male peers. He said that his voice is a source of criticism and teasing from classmates.

Indirect flexible nasoendoscopy performed prior to this evaluation revealed normal vocal fold motion. According to the otolaryngologist's report, small bilateral contact ulcers were noted.

Travis is in good health. He has gone through puberty. No endocrine problems are suspected. He has had no surgeries or trauma to the head or neck. History is negative for reflux symptoms, allergies, and sinusitis. No medications are taken regularly. Fluid intake is moderate, with approximately two caffeinated beverages consumed daily. He denies cigarette and alcohol use.

With regard to stress, Travis stated that he has been having difficulty getting along with his parents. He has discussed this with his school guidance counselor. Travis is the older of three siblings. He is not involved in acting or singing.

EVALUATION
Pitch

Speaking fundamental frequency for /a/ was 218 Hz which exceeds that expected for his gender. Volitional phonation range was from 139-502 Hz, approximately 14 whole notes. Optimal pitch, achieved through throat clearing and hard glottal attack initiation of vowel sounds was estimated at 110-120 Hz. Frequent pitch breaks were heard, as were periods of diplophonia.

Quality

Intermittent mild roughness with accompanying moderate breathiness was noted. Occasional phonation breaks were present.

Loudness

Quiet for a small group setting. Loudness appeared to be controlled to reduce the frequency of pitch breaks. Mean intensity of 71 dB.

Respiration

Shallow, poorly supported breathing observed. Sustained /a/ averaged 9 seconds, which is substantially below normal limits for his age and gender.

Vocal Abuse Behaviors

The following abuses were identified:
- Throat clearing
- Whispering
- Talking at an inappropriately high pitch level

Copyright © 2007 by Mosby, Inc., an affiliate of Elsevier Inc. All rights reserved.

Musculoskeletal Tension

The larynx was elevated, with decreased thyrohyoid space. Travis reported no soreness in the extrinsic laryngeal muscles. Physically depressing the larynx while the client phonated resulted in a lower pitch.

Articulation

No consistent articulation errors were noted. Overall articulator contacts lacked force.

TRIAL THERAPY

It was explained to Travis that he was attempting to maintain a higher-pitched voice, rather than allowing his deeper voice to be used, which interfered with the pitch, quality, and loudness of his voice. Varying facilitative techniques were introduced, all of which he willingly tried, though embarrassment was sometimes expressed. The purpose of each was to lower his pitch to a more optimal one. These techniques included:

- Throat clearing and robust laughing with sustained phonation
- Coughing and simultaneously saying monosyllabic words beginning with vowels
- Hard glottal attack initiation of monosyllabic words beginning with vowels
- Manually lowering his larynx while he phonated

The client demonstrated success with these techniques at a one- to three-syllable word and phrase level. He had limited control at this new pitch level, and frequent pitch breaks occurred. The new voice sounded very different and, initially, undesirable to him.

SUMMARY

This 15-year-old postpubescent male presents with an inappropriately elevated pitch and a breathy, rough voice quality secondary to puberphonia. His voice is a source of embarrassment to him and the focal point for teasing by his peers. Through trial therapy, appropriate pitch was established and maintained for short units of speech. It is felt that when pitch is normalized, loudness and voice quality will return to normal as well. He eventually liked the sound of his new voice, but expressed concern about using it among classmates because of the dramatic difference.

RECOMMENDATIONS

1. Twice-weekly voice therapy sessions for 6 weeks, if indicated.
2. Functional use of "new voice" in all settings and situations on return to school following Christmas break.
3. Share evaluation report and treatment plan with ENT and school SLP.

Long-term Goal

- Travis will speak at a pitch level that is appropriate for his age and gender, in all communication settings, as reported by the client, his parents, and the school SLP.

Short-term Goals

1. Travis will establish an appropriate habitual pitch, through the use of laryngeal massage and vegetative vocal fold functions with 90% consistency.
2. Travis will maintain his targeted habitual pitch from word through conversational levels, in and out of the therapy setting with 80% accuracy as determined through client and clinician charting and report.

Copyright © 2007 by Mosby, Inc., an affiliate of Elsevier Inc. All rights reserved.

VOCAL NODULES AND CYSTS

Most speech-language pathologists, regardless of work setting or population served, will treat a client with vocal nodules. Nodules, also called "singer's nodes" or "screamer's nodes," are caused by vocal abuse and misuse, of which muscle tension or hyperfunction is the outcome. Over time, the area of the vocal fold that receives the greatest impact during vibration (the middle of the membranous portion, also called the *juncture of the anterior third, posterior two thirds*) becomes swollen and irritated, creating mucosal changes. The process of nodule development is somewhat analogous to breaking in new shoes. Initial heel irritation causes swelling and irritation, followed by development of a blister. With increased wear, the blister area becomes a callous. So too with vocal nodules, first localized edema and erythema, then an organized area sometimes called *thickening*, next a reddened, pliable, fluid-filled nodule, followed by a more fibrosed, whitened one. Nodules are typically bilateral, opposing one another on the medial edge of each fold.

Certain populations and occupations appear more predisposed for nodule development, among which includes male children, female adults, cheerleaders, teachers, and singers.

Voice characteristics of speakers with nodules resemble those of MTD. Commonly because of the nodules, glottal closure will be incomplete and hourglass-shaped, causing the voice to have a breathy component. An S/Z ratio greater than one coinciding with the glottal closure pattern, would be expected.[21,70] Additionally, due to the added mass of the vocal nodules, habitual pitch may be decreased, and phonation range may be reduced. Mucosal wave may be reduced in the area surrounding the nodule.

The preferred treatment for vocal nodules is voice therapy that seeks to identify and reduce vocal abuse and misuse, provide vocal hygiene tips, and teach techniques aimed at reducing vocal hyperfunction.[54] Occasionally nodules are removed surgically in situations where voice therapy was unsuccessful in restoring voice to the level desired by the speaker, or on physician recommendation. The unsolved case study of Paul illustrates the latter, where voice therapy was not recommended on diagnosis of vocal nodules by the otolaryngologist.

The case studies included in this book—Nickie, Maddie, and Rachael—are typical of clients with vocal nodules. Maddie and Rachael experienced resolution of their nodules through voice therapy. Nickie discontinued therapy after several sessions, and the status of her vocal folds was unknown.

The trickiest part of treating a client with a diagnosis of nodules is the occasional occurrence of misdiagnosis. Sometimes what is diagnosed as vocal nodules is actually a cyst on one vocal fold and a reactive swelling on the opposing vocal fold. Without stroboscopy, cysts are frequently misdiagnosed as being nodules.[17] Whereas nodules respond and resolve through voice therapy, cysts do not. They require surgical removal. Perceptually, however, speakers with nodules and cysts sound similar: rough, breathy, and strained. The speech-language pathologist treating a client with a diagnosis of nodules should be suspicious when the treatment is appropriate and the client is compliant and the voice still does not improve. In this scenario, the client needs to be reevaluated with stroboscopy to rule out pathologies other than nodules, among which is a cyst. The case study of Robbie illustrates an inaccurate diagnosis of nodules that was actually a cyst on one fold and reactive swelling on the opposing fold.

Copyright © 2007 by Mosby, Inc., an affiliate of Elsevier Inc. All rights reserved.

CASE STUDY 6-1

Vocal Nodules—Adult

 Voice clip #8

BACKGROUND AND REASONS FOR REFERRAL

Nickie, a 21-year-old female, was seen for a voice evaluation upon referral from her roommate, a speech pathology major. The presenting complaints are chronic laryngitis, voice loss, and a low-pitched voice. The client was diagnosed with bilateral vocal fold nodules by her otolaryngologist prior to returning to college from winter break.

HISTORY

According to Nickie, hoarseness developed gradually, with occasional bouts of hoarseness becoming more frequent and lasting longer. She spent the past summer studying abroad and felt that her voice worsened substantially during that time. She attributed this to cigarette use, excessive talking, and inadequate sleep. Since that time, her voice has remained hoarse. She notes these symptoms: throat discomfort and dryness and voice quality that worsens as the day progresses. She describes herself as "very talkative."

History is positive for cigarette smoking, approximately a half pack per day. Caffeine intake is estimated as six beverages per day. Noncaffeinated fluid intake is low, (one or two glasses of water daily). Approximately 15 alcoholic beverages are consumed weekly. Seasonal allergies are experienced and medicated with Clarinex. Advil is taken for frequent headaches. Pepto-Bismol is taken for indigestion and stomach problems, which she attributes to poor diet and an erratic eating schedule.

Nickie is majoring in mass communication. She commented that initially she liked the sound of her husky voice, but now feels that it may interfere with her career.

EVALUATION
Laryngeal Examination

Stroboscopic examination of the larynx revealed bilateral vocal nodules at the anterior 1/3, posterior 2/3 juncture. Additional observations: An hourglass shaped glottic closure pattern; slightly reduced mucosal wave in the area of the lesions; increased glottic and supraglottic compression during phonation.

Pitch

Speaking fundamental frequency was measured at 207 Hz, which is within the normal limits for an adult female of her age. Fundamental frequency pitch range was 155-374 Hz, approximately nine whole tones, which is significantly below normal limits.

Quality

Moderate to severe (4 on a 5-point severity scale) hoarseness and breathiness were heard. Frequent phonation breaks were noted. While reading a 100-word passage, five phonation breaks were heard. Voice quality was consistent throughout the evaluation.

Loudness

Appropriate for a conversational setting (73 dB). She evidenced a loud laugh frequently throughout this session.

Respiration

Normal abdominothoracic breathing patterns were observed. Sustained /a/ of 12 seconds was noted, which is below normal limits for her age and gender. S/Z ratio was 1.2 (18 and 15 seconds, respectively), indicating reduced glottal closure during phonation.

Copyright © 2007 by Mosby, Inc., an affiliate of Elsevier Inc. All rights reserved.

Musculoskeletal Tension

The following signs and symptoms of excessive musculoskeletal tension were noted:

- Frequent headaches, temporomandibular joint (TMJ) pain (more pronounced on the left side), and occasional tinnitus in her left ear.
- Palpation revealed reduced thyrohyoid space, discomfort and tightness of the sternocleidomastoid and trapezius muscles bilaterally.

Vocal Abuse Behaviors

The following abuses were rated on a 1 to 5 scale (5 = the most frequent or severe):

 5—Overall amount of talking; loud talking; phone use
 4—Shouting; yelling; screaming
 3—Throat clearing; talking over noise; whispering

Speech Rate

Excessive when conversing.

TRIAL THERAPY

At the conclusion of this evaluation, the client was counseled on the negative effects of poor vocal hygiene and vocal abuse on vocal fold health. A single vocal abuse was chosen for reduction during the upcoming week. Additionally, the technique of Confidential Voice was taught to Nickie. She will attempt to use it in as many situations as possible, to break her effortful phonation pattern.

SUMMARY

This 21-year-old female presents with bilateral vocal fold nodules secondary to voice abuse and misuse and poor vocal hygiene. Additionally, her lifestyle appears to interfere with vocal and overall health. Voice quality and pitch were most deviant. It was explained to Nickie that voice improvement requires making behavioral changes. It was reinforced that her present voice will likely interfere with her success in a public speaking position. She stated that she is motivated to improve her voice.

RECOMMENDATIONS

1. Participate in voice therapy once weekly for 6 weeks, with continued treatment based on the progress achieved during the 6-week trial.
2. Schedule a physical examination with her internist to discuss stomach concerns and cigarette use.
3. Consult the staff dietician or an athletic trainer at the college for diet, exercise, and relaxation ideas.
4. Stroboscopic examination of the vocal folds if hoarseness does not improve despite client compliance.

Long-term Goal

- Nickie's voice will stay consistent throughout the day with a voice overall severity rating of 2 (mild to moderate) or less as reported by the client and her roommate and rated by the CAPE-V.

Short-term Goals

1. Nickie will reduce vocal abuses by 50% as determined through charting and client report.
2. Nickie will improve vocal hygiene by increasing hydration to 64 oz of noncaffeinated fluids daily; decreasing caffeine to two beverages daily; eliminating smoking; observing three 30-minute voice rest periods daily.
3. Nickie will use voice facilitative techniques to reduce MTD as assessed through posttreatment perceptual and acoustic measures.

Copyright © 2007 by Mosby, Inc., an affiliate of Elsevier Inc. All rights reserved.

CASE STUDY 6-2
Vocal Nodules—Child

 Voice clip #9

BACKGROUND AND REASONS FOR REFERRAL

Maddie, an 8-year-old female, presents with hoarseness of approximately 18 months duration. She was diagnosed with bilateral vocal nodules and referred to this clinic for an evaluation and therapy. Maddie's mother accompanied her to this evaluation, providing additional history information. Maddie's laryngeal examination is located in the diagnostic section of this book, entitled, "Sample Otolaryngology Report".

HISTORY

According to Maddie and her mother, hoarseness and voice breaks, attributed to excessive yelling and screaming, began a year and a half ago, gradually worsening over time. Though Maddie's mother feels that her voice has possibly improved since summer, she described episodes where Maddie is aphonic and uses a great deal of effort to produce an audible voice. While Maddie was not initially bothered by her hoarse voice, she now is hearing comments from her peers.

Medical history appears positive for environmental allergies with symptoms of forceful throat clearing and coughing noted during the fall season. She has no history of asthma symptoms and is not currently on any medication. Birth and developmental history were reported as unremarkable. Maddie had a normal cry as an infant. She has had no surgeries or trauma involving the larynx.

With regard to questions about vocal abuse and misuse, Maddie admitted to screaming frequently throughout her day. She stated that she yells the most during recess despite teacher reminders not to scream. Maddie loves to play outside and is very vocal when playing. She is the youngest of four siblings. She described herself as someone who loves to laugh and talk.

BEHAVIORAL OBSERVATIONS

Maddie presented as a bright, mature child, who was comfortable interacting with adults. She participated in all activities. Throat clearing was heard with frequency during the evaluation session.

EVALUATION
Pitch

Habitual pitch (speaking fundamental frequency) was estimated at 209 Hz, which is in the lower range of normal for an adult female and substantially lower than a female's pitch in her age range. Her phonation range was 182-445 Hz, approximately nine whole tones, which is not within normal limits. It was observed that she speaks near the bottom of her pitch range. Relative average perturbation for /a/ was 2.84, which is not within normal limits (less than 1.00 is WNL), and translates perceptually to vocal hoarseness.

Quality

Moderate to severe breathiness and strain (rated as 4) were heard. Roughness was rated as moderate (3). Frequent phonation breaks were noted. Voice quality was consistent throughout the evaluation, although her voice tended to become less hoarse when she raised her pitch.

Copyright © 2007 by Mosby, Inc., an affiliate of Elsevier Inc. All rights reserved.

NOTES

Loudness

Reduced loudness was noted. Mean loudness for /a/ was 59 dB. The client stated that it is harder to talk soft than it is to talk loud.

Respiration

Normal breathing patterns were observed. S/Z ratio (a comparison of respiration to phonation) was 2.0 (16 and 8 seconds, respectively), indicating incomplete vocal fold closure due to space occupying lesions.

Vocal Abuse Behaviors

The following vocal abuses were identified and rated on a 0 to 5 scale (5 = the most frequent or severe):

    5—Screaming
    4—Shouting or yelling on the playground or outside
    4—Talking excessively
    3—Making funny noises
    3—Coughing; clearing throat
    3—Not drinking enough water

Articulation

No errors noted.

TRIAL THERAPY

At the conclusion of this evaluation, the client and her mother were counseled on the negative effects of vocal overuse and misuse on vocal fold health. Yelling and throat clearing were chosen for reduction during the upcoming week, along with increased hydration. Additionally, the technique of using Confidential Voice to reduce vocal effort and "Silent Cough"[37] to reduce effort of throat clearing, were introduced to Maddie. She will attempt to use these techniques in as many situations as possible, to break her hyperfunctional phonation pattern and throat clear habit.

SUMMARY

This 8-year-old female presents with bilateral vocal fold nodules secondary to voice overuse and misuse. Voice quality, pitch, and loudness are all negatively affected. It was explained to Maddie that voice improvement requires behavioral changes. It was reinforced that her present voice will remain the same if she continues to yell. Maddie seemed motivated to improve her voice. A reward system will be implemented at home.

RECOMMENDATIONS

1. That she participate in voice therapy for minimally six sessions.
2. That her family learns about voice abuse and misuse so that more turn-taking and environmental modifications can be instituted to support Maddie.
3. That she and her classroom teacher determine a "signal" that can be used when Maddie is speaking too loudly, or talking too much, or making noises.
4. That she and her best friend determine a "signal" that can be used on the playground when Maddie is shouting or screaming.
5. That a request be made to allow Maddie to carry a water bottle throughout the school day to increase daily fluid intake.

Long-term Goal

■ Maddie will demonstrate voice improvement and eliminate vocal nodules, by reducing vocal abuse and vocal hyperfunction.

Copyright © 2007 by Mosby, Inc., an affiliate of Elsevier Inc. All rights reserved.

Short-term Goals

1. Maddie will reduce vocal abuses by 50% as determined through charting and client report.
2. Maddie will increase hydration to six glasses of water daily.
3. Maddie will use voice facilitative techniques (chanting, Confidential Voice) to reduce vocal hyperfunction as assessed through perceptual and acoustic measures.
4. Maddie will use the Silent Cough or blowing techniques to reduce throat clearing behaviors by 50%.

Copyright © 2007 by Mosby, Inc., an affiliate of Elsevier Inc. All rights reserved.

CASE STUDY 6-3

Vocal Fold Cyst Misdiagnosed as Vocal Nodules

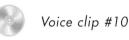 *Voice clip #10*

BACKGROUND AND REASONS FOR REFERRAL

Robbie, an 11-year-old male, was seen for a voice evaluation at this clinic. The chief complaint is hoarseness that impacts his speaking and singing voice. He was diagnosed with bilateral vocal nodules by an otolaryngologist prior to this evaluation, with voice therapy recommended.

HISTORY

According to Robbie and his mother, intermittent hoarseness has been experienced for the past 3 months, first noted in conjunction with his role in a community theatre musical production. Hoarseness worsened following a week at summer camp, which entailed excessive voice abuse. Since that time voice quality has remained consistently poor, prompting a laryngeal examination. Flexible nasolaryngoscopy revealed bilateral vocal nodules. He was asked to observe 3 days of complete voice rest followed by voice therapy.

Robbie is in good health and has had no surgeries or injuries involving the head or neck. History is negative for LPR symptoms; however, a trial course of Prilosec was prescribed by his physician. Robbie has seasonal allergies for which he takes Claritin as needed. His noncaffeinated fluid intake is good. He denies throat pain, but stated that his throat is frequently dry.

Robbie is very active in singing, drama, and sports participation. Additionally he participates in scouts, church activities, and plays a musical instrument. He lives with his mother, father, and a younger sibling. He has never received formal singing training.

EVALUATION (PRETREATMENT)
Pitch

Speaking fundamental frequency was measured at 208 Hz, which is lower than normal for same age boys. Phonation range was 140-393 Hz, approximately 11 whole tones, which is below normal limits. He does not appear to have entered puberty. Frequency perturbation was 1.68.

Quality

Overall voice severity rating was 3 (moderate). Roughness was rated as 2 (mild to moderate) and breathiness was rated as 3 (moderate). Strain was rated as 2 (mild to moderate). Difficulty was observed with phonation onset. Phonation breaks and hard glottal attacks were heard.

Loudness

Appropriate for a small room without background noise. Mean intensity was .71 dB.

Respiration

Maximum phonation duration for /a/ was 13 seconds, which is within normal limits for his age. Ratio for S/Z was 1.1 (15 and 13 seconds, respectively). Normal breathing patterns were observed at rest and during speech.

Vocal Abuse Behaviors

The following behaviors were identified and rated on a 0 to 5 scale (5 indicating most frequent or severe).

    5—Singing
    4—Talking excessively; talking over background noise
    3—Yelling and loud talking associated with play and sports

Copyright © 2007 by Mosby, Inc., an affiliate of Elsevier Inc. All rights reserved.

Articulation

A frontal lisp is noted on /s/ and /z/ in all word positions.

Resonation

Within normal limits.

TRIAL THERAPY

The causes for vocal nodules—voice abuse and voice misuse, and laryngeal muscle hyperfunction were discussed with Robbie and his mother. He was helped to choose two vocal abuse behaviors to reduce during the course of the upcoming week. Additionally he was taught Vocal Function Exercises and given a practice tape for twice daily practices.

SUMMARY

This 11-year-old male presents with a diagnosis of bilateral vocal nodules. His voice is moderately rough, breathy, and effortful with a decreased speaking pitch and a reduced phonation range. It is felt that he has overused and abused his voice while rehearsing for and performing in a musical, with further strain experienced while at camp. It is recommended that he receive weekly voice therapy sessions. Prognosis for voice improvement and nodule resolution depends on Robbie's compliance with voice therapy goals.

RECOMMENDATIONS

1. To refrain from singing other than when performing daily Vocal Function Exercises, until a repeated laryngeal examination is conducted in 6 weeks.
2. To greatly reduce voice abuse, specifically loud talking, talking over noise, and yelling.
3. To observe voice rest for three 20-minute periods during the day, preferably following a period of extended voice use.
4. To improve vocal hygiene by increasing fluids, using a humidifier while sleeping, and continuing with Prilosec.
5. To encourage modifications in voice use at school, extracurricular activities, and at home.
6. To consult with a singing instructor once voice has improved.

Long-term Goal

■ Robbie will experience return of previous vocal function for speaking and singing by reducing voice abuse and misuse and decreasing laryngeal muscle hyperfunction, as determined through perceptual, acoustic, and physiological assessments.

Short-term Goals

1. Robbie will reduce vocal abuses through charting, environmental modification, and a reward system, such that all ratings on the vocal abuse scale are 2 ("sometimes") or less by the completion of therapy.
2. Robbie will reduce vocal hyperfunction through the use of Vocal Function Exercises performed twice daily, minimally 5 days per week, and through Resonant Voice Therapy, as assessed through perceptual, acoustic, and physiological methods.
3. Robbie will improve vocal hygiene through increased hydration and laryngopharyngeal reflux management.

POSTTREATMENT STATUS

Robbie attended 6 weeks of voice therapy. With his family's help, he was very compliant with vocal abuse reduction, vocal hygiene suggestions, and Vocal Function Exercises. At his third session, his speaking fundamental frequency had increased by three semitones; his phonation range had increased by three whole tones (D3-C5) with a break at F4. Maximum phonation duration was 28 seconds, an increase of 15 seconds. His frequency perturbation was 0.55. Perceptually, voice was still rough but improved

Copyright © 2007 by Mosby, Inc., an affiliate of Elsevier Inc. All rights reserved.

in overall quality and strain since the initial evaluation. This was the best voice that Robbie was able to achieve.

Subsequent sessions revealed a decline in Robbie's acoustic and perceptual measures, despite his insistence that he was continuing to monitor voice use and abuse. Videostroboscopy was recommended to examine the structure and vibratory function of his vocal folds.

Examination of his vocal folds revealed a subepithelial cyst on the superior surface of the right vocal fold, with fullness extending to the lateral margin at the middle of the membranous fold. The mucosal wave was reduced at the site of the lesion, and the vibratory amplitude of the right fold was decreased. Slight fullness was observed on the left fold contralateral to the right vocal fold lesion. Vibration was aperiodic. Glottal closure evidenced a posterior glottal chink.

The client and his family were counseled that the cyst would not resolve through therapy alone and that it would require phonosurgery, with postoperative voice therapy. The family was in agreement with this recommendation, and a surgery date was scheduled.

Copyright © 2007 by Mosby, Inc., an affiliate of Elsevier Inc. All rights reserved.

Spasmodic dysphonia (SD) is a neurological voice disorder caused by a lesion of the basal ganglia. It is described as a task-specific focal dystonia,[17] whereby the muscles of the larynx function normally at rest and during vegetative functions but become hypertonic involuntarily during speech, causing muscle spasming heard as phonation and pitch breaks. Depending on which intrinsic muscles are affected, the spasms may be of the abductor type, whereby the vocal folds remain open when they need to close, creating a breathy sound; or of the adductor type, where the folds hyperadduct, causing a squeezed sound. Occasionally both abductor and adductor muscles are affected causing both types of spasms. Sometimes a vocal tremor is heard as well. Its diagnosis stumps speech-language pathologists and otolaryngologists alike due to its strong resemblance to MTD.

The speaker typically reports hoarseness, increased effort or strain associated with voice production, difficulty initiating voice, and intermittent voice breaks. They may report exactly which "letters" (i.e., phonemes) are hardest to say. They describe their voice as unpredictable and inconsistent, noting better voice when they sing, or laugh, or talk at higher pitches. Onset usually is reported as gradual, but occasionally sudden onset is reported. Ongoing stress or a psychological trigger may be reported, occurring prior to the onset of the voice problem, but more typically anxiety is the outcome of the voice problem as the speaker searches for an accurate diagnosis and effective treatment. Frequently, the speaker will have added a muscle tension compensatory response to the SD, making diagnosis even more challenging.

Diagnosis is best accomplished through a team approach including minimally the speech-language pathologist and the otolaryngologist. Flexible nasoendoscopy with videostroboscopy allows the larynx and vocal folds to be visualized, while specific speech tasks designed to elicit the abnormalities are performed. Sometimes, however, the speech-language pathologist is working in a setting where a team approach is not possible. The patient is referred for voice therapy after having had a laryngeal examination and a diagnosis other than spasmodic dysphonia. In both scenarios, trial voice therapy is often the preferred plan of treatment to facilitate an accurate diagnosis and appropriate treatment. For pretreatment and posttreatment efficacy purposes, knowing what tasks and assessment instruments to use and what facilitative techniques to try is of extreme importance. Likewise, astute perceptual skills that aid in identifying deviant voice characteristics such as voice breaks and tremor are a must. The voice evaluation form, Voice Handicap Index,[36] and spasmodic dysphonia diagnostic tasks included in the diagnostic section of this book will guide the speech-language pathologist in the task of differential diagnosis. Likewise, the three case studies and accompanying voice recordings should aid in the diagnostic and trial treatment process.

The most widely used treatment for spasmodic dysphonia is injection of botulinum toxin (also known as *Botox*) into the affected laryngeal muscles.[41] The Botox creates a temporary weakness of the muscles injected, reducing voice strain and spasms. While this improves speech for the majority of patients receiving it, it should be emphasized that it is a treatment and not a cure. Voice therapy in conjunction with Botox treatment can further improve vocal functioning, possibly even extending the time interval between injections.

Copyright © 2007 by Mosby, Inc., an affiliate of Elsevier Inc. All rights reserved.

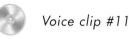

CASE STUDY 7-1

Adductor Spasmodic Dysphonia with Tremor

Voice clip #11

BACKGROUND AND REASONS FOR REFERRAL

Rhonda, a 62-year-old female, was seen for a voice evaluation upon self-referral. The presenting complaints are vocal strain and hoarseness, of 2 years duration.

HISTORY

Various aspects of this client's medical, voice, and social history were vague and contradictory. According to client report, voice problems were experienced for the first time approximately 2 years ago. She could not recall whether the onset was sudden or gradual. Two laryngoscopic examinations were conducted when the dysphonia was first experienced and one year later. According to Rhonda, they were unremarkable with regard to larynx structure and function. In response to the clinician's question, there was no mention of spasmodic dysphonia by the otolaryngologist. No voice therapy has been tried to date. She has worked with a singing instructor on various breathing techniques. She is presently trying self-hypnosis and is practicing various voice techniques at home. Rhonda expressed skepticism toward the medical profession.

Currently, Rhonda reported excessive effort when speaking and a feeling of tightness in her larynx, chest, and mandible. She noted that her breathing has become "mixed up" and consequently interferes with speaking. She reported brief periods of normal voice, occurring on occasional syllables and words and when singing. Laughter also triggers an improved voice. Rhonda stated that her voice problem is interfering with most aspects of her life.

Rhonda described her health as good. She has had no recent surgeries, nor has she had trauma to the head or neck. She reported no family history of neurological disease. She has not noticed any changes in her articulation (although it is labored due to phonation), resonation, motor behavior, or cognition. History is negative for allergies. No symptoms of reflux are reported. She does not smoke nor does she drink caffeinated beverages. Alcohol is consumed occasionally. She has not noticed voice improvement after drinking an alcoholic beverage. Fluid intake is good.

The client was very hesitant to disclose personal information, even her date of birth. When asked questions of a sensitive nature, she became quite defensive, asking why the information was needed. Rhonda communicated through writing for portions of today's evaluation.

EVALUATION
Pitch

Speaking fundamental frequency, measured from sustained vowels was 245 Hz, which is relatively high for a female in her age range. During connected speech, fundamental frequency varied greatly, with easiest phonation at the extremes of her pitch range. Fundamental frequency range was measured at 143-566 Hz, 14 whole notes, which is below the 16- to 24-note normal limit range. A 5 cycle per second (cps) tremor was heard on sustained vowels.

Quality

Severe strained-strangled hoarseness, with intermittent voice breaks was heard. Great difficulty was noted in initiating voice. Oral reading of a 100-word passage required 2.5 minutes (normal speech rate is 160+ words per minute) to complete. Laughter also evidenced a "tight" quality, although much less so than speech. A normal throat clear was noted. When asked to sustain vowels, after the initial difficulty of voice onset, the

Copyright © 2007 by Mosby, Inc., an affiliate of Elsevier Inc. All rights reserved.

strained quality was reduced. Speech intelligibility was greatly impacted by her voice disorder.

Loudness

Excessive strain accompanying phonation interfered with her ability to subtly alter loudness. It volleyed between bursts of loud voice and whispered voice. When sustaining vowel sounds in an easier voice, loudness was appropriate, and she was able to vary loudness.

Respiration

At rest, when not speaking, normal breathing patterns were observed. During speech, Rhonda was observed to speak on both the inhalation and exhalation phases of the cycle. When requested to whisper, thus reducing effort, speech on inhalation continued. When sustaining vowels, phonation on exhalation was sustained maximally for 13 seconds, which approaches normal limits for her age and sex.

Musculoskeletal Tension

Palpation revealed an elevated larynx with a reduced thyrohyoid space. The sternocleidomastoid muscles bilaterally, as well as the larynx, were sensitive to massage. Laryngeal massage was successful in lowering the vertical position of the larynx. No appreciable difference in voice quality was observed following laryngeal massage.

Vocal Abuse Behaviors

None were identified.

Voice Handicap Index

The Voice Handicap Index (VHI) scale, which seeks to assess the level of impact caused by the voice problem within three areas: physical, emotional, and functional, was rated by the client on a 0 to 4 severity scale (0 = never; 4 = always).
Total VHI score: 84/120
   Subscale scores:
   31/40 Physical
   26/40 Functional
   27/40 Emotional

Resonation

Within normal limits.

Articulation

Within normal limits, without dysarthria or apraxia.

TRIAL THERAPY

Trial therapy focused on two goals. The first was developing an awareness of and eliminating speech on inhalation, because this greatly contributed to the bizarreness of Rhonda's speech. A hierarchy was developed: breath practice without speech, correct breath cycles with whisper, and finally correct breath cycles with voiced phonation. By the second diagnostic session, she demonstrated consistent awareness when she spoke on inhalation and was attempting to phonate only on exhalation with fair success. The second goal was conscious control of easy phonation. Yawn–sigh, resonant voice, visual imagery, singing, and sustaining vowels were tried. Resonant voice and singing appeared to foster improved phonation with greatly reduced strain. Improved voice at the word level was noted; however, inconsistency as well as difficulty with voice onset were ongoing problems.

Copyright © 2007 by Mosby, Inc., an affiliate of Elsevier Inc. All rights reserved.

SUMMARY

Rhonda presents with severe dysphonia and voice stoppages that have worsened over 2 years duration. Voice is characterized as strained-strangled, with excessive effort, occurring on both inhalation and exhalation. The voice disorder is significantly impacting functional, physical, and emotional aspects of her life. Laryngoscopic examination performed seemingly near the onset of the voice problem yielded, according to client report, no significant findings. During two diagnostic sessions, many examples of improved voice were heard. Because of the severe strained-strangled quality and tremor noted in Rhonda's voice, a neurological etiology, specifically adductor spasmodic dysphonia, with an additional hyperfunctional compensatory component, is strongly suggested. These findings were discussed with Rhonda, as was her need for further medical evaluation. She expressed a strong desire to try voice therapy before seeking medical evaluation.

RECOMMENDATIONS

1. Receive diagnostic voice therapy for six sessions (two sessions per week).
2. Temporarily reduce the amount of talking in the strained voice by substituting an easy whisper or "chant-type" voice.
3. Refer for psychological counseling.
4. Laryngeal examination via flexible nasoendoscopy and stroboscopy once trust has been established.

Long-term Goals

- Rhonda will develop speech that is intelligible in all conversational speech settings as determined by perceptual assessment and client report.
- Rhonda will improve her perception of herself as a speaker, as determined by a statistically significant decrease in posttreatment scores on the Voice Handicap Index.

Short-term Goals

1. To reduce effortful phonation through the use of voice facilitative techniques such as yawn-sigh, chanting, singing and Resonant Voice Therapy, as assessed through the CAPE-V, yielding perceptual ratings in the moderate range of voice severity.
2. To consistently eliminate phonation on inhalation as determined through perceptual evaluation and client report.
3. To learn and use relaxation techniques, laryngeal massage, visual imagery, and positive self-talk to reduce tension in the upper torso, as determined through observation and client report.

POSTTREATMENT STATUS

Following 6 voice therapy sessions, Rhonda had eliminated phonation on inhalation, and was consistently using humming to initiate voice onset with fair success. She related that she was attempting to talk more as opposed to communicating through writing. Voice stoppages continued to occur with frequency, interfering with intelligibility and prosody. Best voice was achieved when the client sang, during which time speech was fluent once initiated. Carry over into running speech using chanting was not successful. Flexible nasoendoscopy revealed normal vocal fold structure. Hyperadduction of the true vocal folds, and supraglottic constriction were observed with phonation onset, and intermittently throughout the adductor spasmodic dysphonia voice tasks. The client was counseled on her diagnosis of adductor spasmodic dysphonia as well as possible treatment options, of which she was not receptive. Approximately 2 years later, she phoned the author, with a significantly improved voice, announcing proudly that she had recently received her first Botox treatment!

Copyright © 2007 by Mosby, Inc., an affiliate of Elsevier Inc. All rights reserved.

CASE STUDY 7-2

Adductor Spasmodic Dysphonia

 Voice clip #12

BACKGROUND AND REASONS FOR REFERRAL

Leah, a 27-year-old female, was seen for a voice evaluation at this clinic upon referral from her otolaryngologist. The presenting complaints are hoarseness and voice strain of 3 months duration.

HISTORY

According to Leah, she began noticing her voice "cracking" approximately 3 months ago. Subsequently she noted hoarseness and a rapid deterioration of her voice over the course of a few weeks. She consulted with her primary care physician and was prescribed an antibiotic and nasal spray. Voice did not improve, prompting her to consult an otolaryngologist. "Laryngeal inflammation" was reported consistent with laryngitis and laryngopharyngeal reflux. She was prescribed Prilosec for reflux and a steroid for swelling and was advised to have an upper G-I series, which showed no evidence of reflux during the course of the study. Following steroid use, when no voice improvement was noted, Leah consulted another otolaryngologist for flexible videonasoendoscopy and stroboscopy. Results of these examinations revealed normal vocal fold structure, with abnormal function. Severe medial–lateral and moderate anteroposterior vocal fold compression was observed. Amplitude of vibration and mucosal wave were reduced bilaterally. Medial compression of the ventricular folds was observed. A posterior gap was noted during vocal fold vibration. A diagnosis of MTD was given. Voice therapy was recommended.

Leah reports good health. She has seasonal allergies that she treats with antihistamines. She has had no previous voice problems. She does not smoke. Noncaffeinated fluid intake is good. One caffeinated beverage is consumed daily.

Significant medical history includes depression. Current medications include Zoloft. Leah is under the care of a psychiatrist for medication management.

Leah lives with her sister. Current stress includes a new job, for which a great deal of speaking is required, and a sibling with a recent cancer diagnosis.

EVALUATION
Pitch

Fundamental frequency for sustained /a/ was 131 Hz, which is not within normal limits for her age and gender. Optimal pitch (where improved quality was heard) for "uh huh" was 207–308 Hz. There was an absence of pitch inflections. Frequency perturbation was 4.11, which greatly exceeds normal limits, and correlates perceptually with excessive vocal roughness.

Quality

Overall voice severity was rated as 4 (moderate to severe). Consistent roughness resembling effortful glottal fry was rated as 4 (moderate to severe), strain as 3 (moderate), and breathiness as 1 (mild). No voice spasms were heard during the reading or speech sample. Voice quality remained consistent throughout all tasks, with poorer quality and rapid pulsing-type voice flutter noted on sustained vowels. The sound of Leah's throat clear, cough, and laugh was discrepant from her speaking voice, having a clearer, stronger sound.

Loudness

Inadequate for a small group setting. Voice quality worsened when attempts were made to increase loudness.

Copyright © 2007 by Mosby, Inc., an affiliate of Elsevier Inc. All rights reserved.

Respiration

Normal abdominothoracic breathing patterns were observed. Breath patterns reflected the client's anxiety regarding her voice. Maximum phonation duration (MPD) for /a/ averaged 15 seconds, which approaches normal limits.

Musculoskeletal Tension

Elevated larynx with reduced thyrohyoid space.

Vocal Abuse Behaviors

The following vocal abuses were reported as excessive by the client:

>   Excessive use of speaking voice while working
>   Talking loudly and in the presence of noise
>   Throat clearing (attempts to improve voice quality)

Voice Handicap Index

The Voice Handicap Index (VHI) scale, which seeks to assess the level of impact caused by the voice problem within three areas: physical, emotional, and functional, was rated by the client on a 0 to 4 severity scale (0 = never; 4 = always).
Total VHI score: 76/120

>   *Subscale scores:*
>   27/40 Physical
>   23/40 Functional
>   26/40 Emotional

Resonation

Within normal limits.

Articulation

Within normal limits without dysarthria.

TRIAL THERAPY

Improved voice was achieved through the use of laryngeal massage in conjunction with yawn-sigh, glissandos, use of "um hum," and voicing following laughter. Best voice was achieved with "um hum," and using this to initiate speech, Leah phonated vowels and counted. Clear voice was maintained when counting, grouping two numbers together, using "um hum" to initiate each number group. There was no carryover heard after trial therapy. At the conclusion of this evaluation, the client was counseled on the negative effects of vocal abuse and misuse on vocal fold health.

SUMMARY

Leah presents with a diagnosis of MTD of 3 months duration. She feels that her voice disorder is greatly impacting her life at functional, physical, and emotional levels. She is very concerned about her voice and expresses a strong desire for improvement.

Leah's voice disorder negatively affects pitch, quality, and loudness. Her speaking voice is best described as effortful glottal fry, which allows her to communicate provided she maintains this controlled manner of voicing. Sustained vowel production was more difficult, evidencing greater variation in roughness and pitch, with fluctuating increased tightness heard, although no actual voice stoppages. Trial therapy was successful in achieving good voice with regard to improved quality at an appropriate pitch. It could be maintained for only two to three words or syllables at a time. This was encouraging to the client.

RECOMMENDATIONS

1. Six sessions of trial voice therapy for differential diagnostic and treatment purposes.
2. Discussion of the case with the referring otolaryngologist.

Copyright © 2007 by Mosby, Inc., an affiliate of Elsevier Inc. All rights reserved.

3. Periodic perceptual, acoustic, and videostroboscopic evaluation to assess and document voice status and vocal fold function during the therapy process.

4. Exploration of whether a psychogenic component is part of this voice disorder.

Long-term Goal

■ Leah will establish and maintain phonation that is within normal limits for her age and gender and allows for successful communication within her job.

Short-term Goal

■ Leah will use voice facilitative techniques (laryngeal massage, yawn-sigh, humming, chanting, etc.) to reduce MTD, as assessed through perceptual, acoustic and videostroboscopic methods.

POSTTREATMENT STATUS

After 4 weeks of twice weekly voice therapy sessions, Leah sought the expertise of an otolaryngologist highly skilled in diagnosing laryngeal problems. Through voice therapy, she was able to produce phrases with a clear voice provided she used "uh huh" to initiate each phrase. She practiced minimally an hour each day and attempted to use her target voice whenever possible at work. She never experienced success beyond a phrase level. The strained, effortful voice would always return. The frustration of trying to work in a public setting with a significant voice disorder was overwhelming because of functional, physical, and emotional consequences.

The otolaryngologist diagnosed her with early adductor spasmodic dysphonia and recommended Botox treatment. She was treated with Botox injections, resulting in improved voice and greater success in performing tasks requiring voice. Administration of the Voice Handicap Index (VHI) after Leah had had several courses of Botox therapy revealed that despite improved voice, she continued to feel handicapped by her voice. Prior to Botox treatment, her total VHI score was 76 out of a possible 120 points. Following Botox treatment, the total VHI score was 54, indicating a 22 point reduction, which is a statistically significant improvement, yet still indicative of voice dissatisfaction.

Copyright © 2007 by Mosby, Inc., an affiliate of Elsevier Inc. All rights reserved.

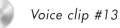

CASE STUDY 7-3

Mixed Abductor/Adductor Spasmodic Dysphonia

Voice clip #13

BACKGROUND AND REASONS FOR REFERRAL

Emma, a 26-year-old wife, mother, and teacher, was seen for a voice evaluation at this clinic upon referral from her otolaryngologist. The presenting complaints are hoarseness and voice breaks of 1 year duration.

HISTORY

According to Emma, voice problems began gradually. Initially it was attributed to postnasal drip; however, treatment for chronic sinusitis did not improve her voice. She notes that her voice is consistent throughout the day, but reports that some days are worse than others. Her voice often feels "strained" and "tired." The hoarseness and voice breaks interfere with her being understood when speaking on the phone. She finds it particularly hard to say /t/, /f/, and /k/ sounds. She finds her voice debilitating both at home and at work.

Emma has had her larynx examined twice through nasoendoscopy by an otolaryngologist since onset of voice problems. The examination was remarkable for LPR; however, no other significant findings were reported. According to Emma, she was asked to phonate /i/ only, with no other laryngeal or phonation gestures requested.

History is negative for cigarette and alcohol use. Caffeine intake is low. Reflux symptoms are reported and are being treated with Prilosec and behavioral management. Oral contraceptives are used. There has been no reported trauma involving the head or neck. Nasal septum surgical repair was done 5 months before this evaluation. There have been no other surgeries. No family history of voice or neurological problems is reported. Emma has not observed any change in her articulation, resonance, or motor abilities.

Emma described herself as a quiet, shy person who is an overachiever and sets high standards for herself. Ongoing stress includes balancing home and work demands.

EVALUATION
Pitch

Fundamental frequency for sustained /a/ was 220 Hz. Perceptually, habitual speaking pitch is within the lower range of normal for age and gender (195 Hz). Fundamental frequency phonation range was 146-523 Hz, approximately 15 whole tones. There was no evidence of tremor.

Quality

Overall voice severity was rated as 3 (moderate). Roughness was rated as 2, and strain as 2 (mild to moderate). Most noticeable were the frequent voice breaks, predominantly of the abductor type, following voiceless and voiced consonants. While reading the "Rainbow Passage,"[24] consisting of 100 words, 18 voice breaks were heard. Voice onset difficulties were heard when phonating sustained vowels. The sound of Emma's laugh was discrepant from her speaking voice, having a clearer, stronger sound.

Loudness

Adequate for a small group setting with no background noise. When increased loudness was demonstrated, voice quality worsened.

Respiration

Normal abdominothoracic breathing patterns were observed. Maximum phonation duration (MPD) for /a/ averaged 11 seconds, which is not within normal limits.

Copyright © 2007 by Mosby, Inc., an affiliate of Elsevier Inc. All rights reserved.

Musculoskeletal Tension

Prominent strap muscles were observed during phonation. Pain was not reported with laryngeal palpation.

Vocal Abuse Behaviors

The following vocal abuse was reported as excessive by the client:
   Throat clearing

Voice Handicap Index

The Voice Handicap Index (VHI) scale, which seeks to assess the level of impact caused by the voice problem within three areas: physical, emotional, and functional, was rated by the client on a 0 to 4 severity scale (0 = never; 4 = always).
Total VHI score: 70/120
   Subscale scores:
   24/40 Physical
   24/40 Functional
   22/40 Emotional

Resonation

Within normal limits.

Articulation

Within normal limits without dysarthria.

TRIAL THERAPY

Using the voice facilitative techniques of Resonant Voice Therapy (RVT) and chanting, Emma demonstrated improved voice with reduced voice breaks for short segments of automatic speech (counting and days of the week). Though she was unable to carry over this voice into other speech contexts, it was felt that this had positive prognostic value.

SUMMARY

Emma presents with mild to moderate roughness, breathiness, and strain; reduced loudness, and voice breaks, most often of the abductor type, of 1 year duration. Laryngeal examination revealed presence of reflux. Emma is very motivated to understand the cause of her voice disorder, and to improve her voice. Trial therapy during this evaluation demonstrated reduced hoarseness and less voice breaks in very structured speech tasks. At the conclusion of the evaluation, Emma was counseled on the possible etiologies responsible for the characteristics heard in her voice. Information about MTD and spasmodic dysphonia was provided.

RECOMMENDATIONS

It was recommended that Emma participate in diagnostic voice therapy for several sessions to allow adequate time to determine the nature of her voice problem and her responsiveness to therapy. It was also recommended that the client receive flexible nasoendoscopy and stroboscopy from an otolaryngologist who has extensive experience in diagnosing and treating voice and laryngeal disorders of neurogenic etiology. The client was in agreement with these recommendations.

Long-term Goal

■ Emma will establish and maintain voice that has reduced roughness and voice breaks and allows successful communication both at home and at work.

Short-term Goals

1. The client will reduce voice breaks by 75% through the use of voice facilitative techniques, as assessed through pretreatment and posttreatment recordings of the CAPE-V and "Rainbow Passage."

Copyright © 2007 by Mosby, Inc., an affiliate of Elsevier Inc. All rights reserved.

2. The client will experience improvement in the physical, functional and emotional ratings of her voice disorder as evidenced by an 18-point or greater reduction on the Voice Handicap Index.

3. The client will demonstrate reduced reflux symptoms through behavioral and medication intervention as evidenced by pretreatment and posttreatment scores on the Reflux Symptom Index.

POSTTREATMENT STATUS

Following four voice therapy sessions, there was no improvement noted in Emma's overall voice rating. When re-reading the "Rainbow Passage," 16 predominantly abductor voice breaks were heard, as compared to 18 noted during the initial evaluation. Slower voice onset times were noted as compared with 4 weeks previously. The Voice Handicap Index revealed a 2-point increase as compared with the initial evaluation. Further investigation by an otolaryngologist and neurologist was recommended. The otolaryngologist's findings are reported in the diagnostic section of this book.

Copyright © 2007 by Mosby, Inc., an affiliate of Elsevier Inc. All rights reserved.

A full discussion of vocal fold paralysis is beyond the scope of this book because of its various presentations, which are determined by the site of the lesion. Included in the diagnostic section of this book are several resources that will assist the speech-language pathologist in developing a better understanding of the neuroanatomy and physiology of the vagus nerve, which innervates the intrinsic laryngeal muscles. A diagram is included of the vagus nerve[11] that depicts it from its origin in the medulla; illustrated are the nerve branches that innervate muscles for velopharyngeal competence (pharyngeal branch), pitch change, and laryngeal sensation (superior laryngeal branch [SLN]) and vocal fold abduction and adduction (recurrent laryngeal branch [RLN]). Noting the asymmetrical course of the left and right recurrent laryngeal nerves and how the left RLN wraps around the aorta aids the SLP in understanding why left RLN paralyses occur with increased frequency. Included also is a flow chart adapted from the Aronson text[11] that clarifies the location of the site of lesion, the muscle(s) affected, and the associated voice (and resonance) problems. Finally, the Netsell and Boone diagram[50] showing the areas within the vocal tract where air is valved for voice and speech production is extremely helpful in diagnosing the various components in dysarthric speech and the associated "valve(s)" that are functioning abnormally. This diagram functions as a treatment model as well, aiding the clinician in determining areas of greatest motor abnormality. Once determined, treatment can target areas of weakness to strengthen, or areas of strength to compensate for weaker ones.

Three case studies of vocal fold paralysis are included in this section of the book; an additional case study is presented in the "Unsolved Case Studies" section. Tina and Jean presented with unilateral recurrent laryngeal nerve paralysis, whereas Steve had a paralysis involving the pharyngeal, superior laryngeal, and recurrent laryngeal branches of the vagus nerve secondary to a brainstem CVA. For two of the clients, a return of nerve and associated muscle function was experienced. Whereas for Jean, a surgical procedure called *thyroplasty* was performed to assist her in closing her glottis for better voice and swallowing.

Because adductor paralysis is seen more often by the SLP than abductor paralysis, this discussion focuses on adductor paralysis.

There are multiple causes for vocal fold paralysis, trauma and disease comprising the main two categories. When the cause of the paralysis is unknown, it is called *idiopathic*. When the paralysis was caused unintentionally, secondary to another procedure, such as during cardiac bypass surgery or thyroidectomy, it is called *iatrogenic*.

Typically (depending on the position of the paralyzed fold), the speaker will experience a breathy, hoarse voice; a feeling of running out of air while speaking; an inability to talk loudly, and dysphagia. A speaker may have respiratory complaints unassociated with speech. These symptoms indicate that the vocal folds are not meeting and closing in the midline, thereby allowing some degree of glottal incompetence.

Several medical, surgical treatment options are available for adductor paralysis. Generally a waiting period of 6 months or greater is allowed to pass, during which time no permanent solution to the paralysis is undertaken. During this time, it is hoped that the nerve will regain function spontaneously, allowing the vocal fold to resume normal function. If voice and swallowing function are significantly impaired during this waiting period, then an augmentation procedure may be performed, injecting material (such as gel foam that is gradually absorbed by the larynx) into the paralyzed fold, thereby giving it added mass to aid glottal closure.

Copyright © 2007 by Mosby, Inc., an affiliate of Elsevier Inc. All rights reserved.

NOTES

If the paralysis appears permanent, additional medical and surgical procedures are possible. They include augmentation with a substance such as collagen; thyroplasty, a surgical procedure that medializes the paralyzed fold through inserting a wedge through a surgically created window in the side of the thyroid cartilage; arytenoid adduction to approximate the folds; and reinnervation of the paralyzed vocal fold through a nerve crossover procedure, thereby reestablishing muscle bulk and tone.

Voice therapy is effective in the treatment of vocal cord paralysis from a direct treatment approach, aimed at improving glottal closure; or from a compensatory approach aimed at improving communication. The speech-language pathologist's role with the four paralysis case studies presented in this book varied for each speaker. Facilitative techniques targeting glottal closure appeared effective in aiding return of function for Steve. Therapy for Jean after thyroplasty aided in establishing her best voice, in part through undoing habituated muscle tension patterns. Tina's paralysis had probably resolved by the time she came for therapy, but other than breath control, she had continued using the "paralysis voice." Finally Evan, having bilateral paralysis, was best helped by teaching him to intentionally vibrate his supraglottic structures, giving him a more serviceable voice.

Copyright © 2007 by Mosby, Inc., an affiliate of Elsevier Inc. All rights reserved.

CASE STUDY 8-1

Unilateral Recurrent Laryngeal Nerve Paralysis Following Thyroplasty

 Voice clip #14

BACKGROUND AND REASONS FOR REFERRAL

Jean, a 43-year-old wife and mother, was seen for a voice evaluation at this clinic upon referral from her otolaryngologist. She had recently undergone thyroplasty to medialize her left vocal fold and is presently concerned about the residual hoarse quality of her voice.

HISTORY

Jean has experienced voice weakness for the past 18 months secondary to idiopathic left recurrent nerve paralysis. During this time, she received no medical treatment or voice therapy. The paralyzed vocal fold did not regain function. When accompanying her husband to a medical appointment with an otolaryngologist, the otolaryngologist suggested that Jean's voice could be improved through thyroplasty, a surgical technique to move the paralyzed fold closer toward the midline of the glottis for improved glottal closure, positively influencing voice and swallowing. Since having the surgery, Jean has noted gradual voice improvement and reduced effort needed to speak. She states that her voice fatigues with continued use and that her larynx feels sore by evening. She notes improvement with swallowing and also with breathing during exercise, stating that before the surgery she always "lost her air."

Jean has a positive medical history of allergies to dust and molds. She suffers occasional migraines. She is followed by a neurologist for Barlow's syndrome. She takes the following medications: Tofranil, Xanax, Inderal, and Prozac. History is negative for cigarette and alcohol use. Caffeine intake is low. Overall fluid intake is high. Reflux symptoms are denied.

Jean has five children ranging in age from 5 to 14 years. Home and family demands require frequent voice use, often at above average loudness levels. Ongoing stress includes her husband's inability to find work, and lack of medical insurance. Before having voice problems she enjoyed singing and performed with her sister for church-related singing engagements.

LARYNGEAL EXAMINATION

Jean's larynx was examined transnasally using a flexible laryngoscope. Stroboscopy was not available. The left vocal fold was noted to be slightly bowed but without swelling. The left false vocal fold was hypertrophied and demonstrated medial compression, at times impeding the view of the left true fold. There was a slight irritation of the right arytenoid caused by the left arytenoid pressing against it when the folds are adducted. Vertical plane of the two vocal folds appeared symmetrical; however, without stroboscopy this could not easily be determined.

EVALUATION
Pitch

Fundamental frequency for sustained /a/ was 208 Hz. Perceptually, pitch is within the lower range of normal for age and gender. Fundamental frequency phonation range was 182-604 Hz, approximately 12 and ½ whole tones, which is not within normal limits. Diplophonia was intermittently present and increased when attempting to talk louder. A frequency tremor was heard on sustained vowels.

Copyright © 2007 by Mosby, Inc., an affiliate of Elsevier Inc. All rights reserved.

Quality

Overall voice severity was rated as 2 (mild to moderate). Roughness and breathiness were rated as 2 (mild to moderate) for speech and 3 (moderate) for sustained vowels. Strain was rated as 2 (mild to moderate). When talking in a louder voice, roughness, breathiness, diplophonia, and strain increased. Best vocal quality was achieved when Jean produced sustained vowels with a singing style. Cough and throat clear were strong.

Loudness

Jean's voice was audible for a small group setting with no background noise, which differs considerably from her home environment.

Respiration

Normal abdominothoracic breathing patterns were observed. Intermittently audible inspiration was noted but without stridor. Maximum phonation duration for /a/ averaged 14 seconds, which approaches normal limits for her age and gender. S/Z ratio was 1.4 (26 and 18 seconds, respectively), which suggests reduced glottal closure for phonation. Breath management with regard to phrasing was evaluated through reading of the "Rainbow Passage." The average number of syllables per breath was 12.2, with a range of 3 to 18 syllables, which is reduced when compared to speakers without vocal fold motion impairment.

Musculoskeletal Tension

Excessive musculoskeletal tension was reported as manifesting in headaches and temporomandibular joint pain (TMJ).

Vocal Abuse Behaviors

The following vocal abuses were rated on a 1 to 5 scale with 5 being most frequent or severe.

    5—Throat clearing
    4—Talking loudly; phone use
    3—Talking excessively, talking over noise, whispering

Voice Handicap Index

The Voice Handicap Index (VHI) scale, which seeks to assess the level of impact caused by the voice problem within three areas: physical, emotional, and functional, was rated by the client on a 0 to 4 severity scale (0 = never; 4 = always).
Total VHI score: 63/120
    Subscale scores:
    21/40 Physical
    30/40 Functional
    12/40 Emotional
    These results suggest that overall Jean is feeling positive toward herself as a speaker, but is limited by her voice performance physically and, to a greater extent, functionally.

Resonation

Within normal limits.

Articulation

Within normal limits without dysarthria.

TRIAL THERAPY

Vocal Function Exercises, a group of systematic laryngeal phonatory exercises designed to strengthen and rebalance the muscles of the larynx and the overall vocal system, were introduced and taught to the client. An audiotape of the exercises was given to Jean for twice daily practice, along with a chart on which to plot her performance.

Copyright © 2007 by Mosby, Inc., an affiliate of Elsevier Inc. All rights reserved.

SUMMARY

Jean presents with mild to moderate residual roughness, breathiness, and diplophonia secondary to vocal fold medialization surgery, for vocal fold paralysis. The client enjoyed singing before the onset of vocal fold paralysis and would like to be able to sing again. She has five children, which requires her to talk often and loudly. Additionally, she is experiencing a great deal of stress, which she feels negatively impacts her emotional status and her voice. She expressed disappointment regarding the outcome of her surgery, having hoped she would experience a return of her preparalysis voice.

RECOMMENDATIONS

It was recommended that Jean participate in voice therapy to target the deviant aspects of her voice. It was felt that some of the negative characteristics of her voice, such as breath control for phrasing, and muscle effort associated with phonation may be habitual responses to vocal fold paralysis, which can now be unlearned because glottal closure has improved. It was explained to the client that the paralyzed vocal fold, although now being in a better position for vibration and closure, still does not possess the movement and muscle tone that it had before paralysis. Thus expecting a return of the preparalysis voice may not be a realistic goal.

Additional recommendations included:

1. Videostroboscopic examination of vocal fold vibration once medical insurance is obtained.
2. Reduction of vocal abuses; substituting less effortful voice and methods of instruction and discipline that are less reliant on voice.
3. Investigation of counseling services through her church to help with stress and depression management.

Long-term Goal

▪ Jean will maintain a voice that allows her to be successful at home with her family with normal levels of background noise as assessed through client and family report.

Short-term Goals

1. The client will reduce vocal effort and lengthen phrasing through the use of Vocal Function Exercises, as assessed through prerecording and postrecording of the "Rainbow Passage" and maximum phonation duration for /a/ that approximates that of sustained /s/.
2. The client will experience improvement in the physical and functional aspects of her voice as evidenced by a significant reduction of her score on the VHI.

POSTTREATMENT STATUS

After eight voice therapy sessions, it appears that Jean's voice has plateaued. Considerable progress has been achieved through voice therapy, with short-term and long-term goals met.

Pitch

Habitual pitch is unchanged since the initial evaluation. Pitch range, however, has increased by two whole tones. Diplophonia continues to be heard at high loudness levels.

Quality

Mild roughness noted, but reduced breathiness and strain.

Loudness

She continues to be a quiet speaker, but states that she can increase her loudness to call her children without feeling the need to strain. Mean intensity was 70 dB.

Copyright © 2007 by Mosby, Inc., an affiliate of Elsevier Inc. All rights reserved.

Respiration

Normal phrasing has been achieved. Maximum phonation duration for /a/ sustained at G4 (390 Hz) is 30 seconds.

Vocal Abuse Behaviors

The following vocal abuses were reported as excessive by the client:
Talking excessively
Talking in the presence of noise
Throat clearing

Voice Handicap Index

An overall reduction (indicative of improvement) on the VHI score was noted. Jean's total score was 44/120 points, reflecting a 19-point improvement since it was first administered. Her score improved by 13 points with regard to the functional impact of her voice disorder and 6 points with regard to the physical impact, suggesting that voice has improved and/or she has become better adjusted to her voice.

SINGING

- Jean has begun singing at home with her daughters and feels encouraged regarding her singing voice.

Copyright © 2007 by Mosby, Inc., an affiliate of Elsevier Inc. All rights reserved.

CASE STUDY 8-2
Vocal Cord Paralysis

 Voice clip #15

BACKGROUND AND REASONS FOR REFERRAL

Steve, a 47-year-old business owner, was referred for a voice evaluation by the speech-language pathologist at the facility where he was hospitalized for a stroke 4 months prior to this evaluation. He is presently concerned about the breathy quality of his voice.

HISTORY

Steve suffered a brainstem cerebrovascular accident (CVA) 4 months before this voice evaluation. Immediately after the CVA, he noted these symptoms: a hoarse, breathy voice, a right-sided facial weakness, and difficulty drinking liquids and eating hard solid foods without aspirating. A neurological evaluation determined that the stroke had affected cranial nerves IX, X, XI, XII. Laryngeal imaging revealed a right vocal fold adductor paralysis. A swallowing study diagnosed moderate dysphagia. Dysarthric articulation also was perceived.

Steve had intensive dysphagia therapy while hospitalized. Presently, using the swallowing techniques taught, Steve considers his swallowing to approximate normal, with only occasional problems with thin liquids and hard, dry foods such as pork chops. Upon completion of dysphagia treatment, Steve began voice therapy at the hospital. It was recommended that he seek the services of this clinician for further evaluation and treatment of his voice. No surgical or medical interventions were tried.

Medical history is positive for migraine headaches and hypertension, which are treated with prescription medications. The client experienced anxiety and depression subsequent to his illness. Steve has not had any previous voice problems. He was not intubated during this hospitalization. He does not smoke cigarettes. Alcohol intake is minimal.

With regard to language and cognition, Steve feels that he is not quite "as sharp" as he was before the CVA. He says that he tires more easily and when fatigued has more difficulty retrieving words, following conversations, and remembering details. He has returned to work on a limited basis, but because of his voice, he has had difficulty talking on the telephone, which is vital to his job. Steve has no motor weaknesses in his extremities. He has resumed driving. He is married and has three children, ranging in age from 16 to 2 years old.

EVALUATION VOICE
Laryngoscopy

Video endoscopy revealed paralysis of the right fold in the paramedian position. The fold appeared shortened and flaccid. An absence of arytenoid motion was seen with attempted phonation.

Pitch

Habitual speaking fundamental frequency was estimated at 119 Hz, which is within normal limits for his age and sex. Fundamental frequency pitch range was 85-306 Hz, approximately 13 whole tones, which is not within normal limits. Diplophonia was heard on sustained vowels and connected speech. At a higher pitch, diplophonia ceased, and a single clearer voice was heard. Frequency perturbation was 4.36, which greatly exceeds normal limits and perceptually correlates with vocal hoarseness.

Quality

Severe breathiness with accompanying moderate roughness was heard. Strain accompanied phonation. Dysphonia was consistent throughout the evaluation. Cough and throat clear were weak sounding.

Copyright © 2007 by Mosby, Inc., an affiliate of Elsevier Inc. All rights reserved.

NOTES

Loudness

Audible in the treatment room with no competing background noise. When attempting to increase loudness, the number of syllables that could be phonated on a single exhalation was significantly shortened and vocal effort increased.

Respiration

Breathing was audible on inhalation. Maximum phonation duration for /a/ was 4 seconds, which is significantly below the mean for age and gender. S/Z ratio was 2.2 (14 and 6 seconds, respectively), which strongly suggests inadequate glottal valving during phonation. This was also observed in connected speech through shortened phrases and increased breaths. Reading the first two paragraphs of the "Rainbow Passage," containing 127 syllables, required 18 breaths, with an average of 7 syllables per breath.

Voice Handicap Index

The Voice Handicap Index (VHI) scale, which seeks to assess the level of impact caused by the voice problem within three areas: physical, emotional, and functional, was rated by the client on a 0 to 4 severity scale (0 = never; 4 = always).

> Total VHI score: 74/120
> *Subscale scores:*
> 25/40 Physical
> 29/40 Functional
> 20/40 Emotional

Resonation

Mild hypernasality perceived.

EVALUATION—ORAL MOTOR

Lip puckering and retraction appeared within normal limits. Steve's tongue deviated to the left side at rest and deviated to the right during protrusion and speech movements. The uvula at rest also deviated to the right. A gag reflex was not triggered when touching the posterior tongue, faucial arches, or pharynx. Observation of the soft palate, when asked to say /a/, revealed slight asymmetry with reduced elevation on the right side. Steve reported equal bilateral sensation to touch for the lips, tongue, and palate.

Diadochokinetic rates were obtained from the Verbal Agility Subtest of the Boston Diagnostic Aphasia Examination (BDAE),[28] which required rapid, precise repetition of multisyllabic words and phrases using phonemic combinations that increase in complexity. Reduced articulation precision and slowed rate were observed, especially for lingual sounds. Extreme vocal breathiness and reduced ability to sustain sound made this task very challenging, negatively influencing the results.

EVALUATION—LANGUAGE

The BDAE, Revised Token Test (RTT)[44] and Boston Naming Test (BNT)[37] were administered. Although occasional errors were observed, none of the tests revealed an aphasic deficit. On the BDAE, all subtest scores except that for Oral Agility fell in the 90th to 100th percentile. Only four errors occurred on the RTT, with all four being confusion of color, shape, or size words, as opposed to those of syntactic complexity. On the BNT, 55 of the 60 words were named without cueing (54.4 was the average score for normal adults in his age range).

EVALUATION—HEARING

Results of pure tone, audiological assessment, and word recognition testing were within normal limits bilaterally.

Copyright © 2007 by Mosby, Inc., an affiliate of Elsevier Inc. All rights reserved.

TRIAL THERAPY

The following facilitative techniques were tried: isometric (pushing) exercises, altering head position, and pitch glides. Best voice with reduced hyperfunction was achieved at higher pitches using downward pitch glides starting in a falsetto range.

SUMMARY

After a brainstem CVA, Steve presented with dysphagia and voice and speech problems. His language test scores were within normal limits, although clinically, Steve notes some areas of weakness that increase when he is tired. He has had extensive dysphagia therapy and feels that with conscious monitoring his swallowing is no longer problematic. He has returned to work but is experiencing frustration regarding communication because of his voice. His voice is breathy and hoarse with reduced loudness and shortened phrase lengths, secondary to unilateral vocal fold paralysis. Talking is effortful for him, which causes his voice to fatigue with increased use. His resonation appears to be mildly hypernasal, and his articulation lacks the precision that it had before the CVA. Perceptually, his voice is the most deviant feature of his dysarthria. Producing a stronger voice at higher pitches during this evaluation was encouraging to Steve. This in addition to time since onset of CVA and improved swallowing function are positve prognastic indicators.

RECOMMENDATIONS

The following recommendations were given:
1. Participate in a trial period of voice therapy.
2. Laryngeal imaging with stroboscopy to assess vocal fold structure and function.
3. Observe good vocal hygiene; prioritize voice use; purchase a voice amplification system.
4. Learn and practice Vocal Function Exercises twice daily to improve vocal fold functioning, while reducing hyperfunction.
5. Laryngeal EMG studies if no progress is experienced after 6 months.

Long-term Goal

- Steve will develop the best voice possible using facilitative techniques to enhance glottal closure, as determined through ongoing perceptual, acoustic, aerodynamic, and physiological assessments.

Short-term Goals

1. To eliminate all unnecessary vocal abuse and employ environmental modifications such as voice amplification and listener positioning as determined through client report.
2. To use therapy techniques such as Vocal Function Exercises, glissandos, laryngeal isometrics, head positioning, and hard glottal attack initiation to improve glottal closure and facilitate improved voice.

Copyright © 2007 by Mosby, Inc., an affiliate of Elsevier Inc. All rights reserved.

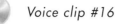

CASE STUDY 8-3

Unilateral Recurrent Laryngeal Nerve Paralysis

Voice clip #16

BACKGROUND AND REASONS FOR REFERRAL

Tina, a 35-year-old female office manager, presented for a voice evaluation. She had a diagnosis of a left recurrent laryngeal nerve paralysis of approximately 7 months duration. She previously received short-term voice therapy at another facility.

HISTORY

According to medical and client report, a fall was sustained that resulted in a diagnosis of chronic regional pain syndrome in the left upper extremity. Subsequently, she received several nerve block procedures in the area of the cervical vertebrae. After the last nerve block, Tina experienced a hoarse, breathy voice. A left recurrent laryngeal nerve paralysis was diagnosed through flexible nasoendoscopy and confirmed by a computed tomography (CT) scan. A subsequent diagnostic work-up ruled out a vagus nerve tumor and lower airway disease as possible etiologies for the paralysis. Speech therapy was recommended but discontinued after four sessions when no progress was achieved.

The client was examined by another otolaryngologist for the purpose of determining worker's compensation benefits 2 weeks before this voice evaluation. Using a flexible scope, the left vocal fold and arytenoid cartilage were reported to have full movement. A large posterior glottal chink was observed with vocal fold adduction. A strong throat clear was heard, despite a breathy, weak speaking voice. Tina was diagnosed with a functional voice disorder. Voice therapy was recommended.

At the time of this evaluation, Tina was convinced that her vocal cord was still paralyzed because her voice had not changed over the past 7 months. She stated that she was unable to perform her work duties or to parent effectively with her current voice status.

Tina does not smoke cigarettes or drink alcohol. Noncaffeinated fluid intake is good. She denies swallowing problems but has lost 10 pounds since her accident. She has not had previous voice problems. She reports no concerns regarding her hearing acuity.

EVALUATION
Pitch

Speaking fundamental frequency for sustained /a/ was 198 Hz, which is low for same age females. Fundamental frequency phonation range was from 185-262 Hz, approximately seven semitones (4 and 1/2 notes), which is not within normal limits. An absence of pitch inflections was noted.

Quality

Mild to moderate roughness (rating of 2) with moderate to severe breathiness (rating of 4) and moderate strain (rating of 3) were perceived. Sustained vowels evidenced intermittent aphonic breaks. Spontaneous speech quality was superior to vowel prolongation.

Loudness

Adequate for a small, quiet environment. The client was unable to increase loudness when requested to do so.

Respiration

Maximum phonation duration for /a/ was 5 seconds, which is not within normal limits. S/Z ratio was 1.5 (12 and 8 seconds, respectively), which suggests reduced glottal

Copyright © 2007 by Mosby, Inc., an affiliate of Elsevier Inc. All rights reserved.

closure for phonation. Breath control for phrasing was reduced but inconsistent, with more frequent breaths taken when reading as compared to conversing. No audible inspiration or stridor was heard.

Vocal Abuse Behaviors

The following were identified and rated on a 1 to 5 scale, with 5 being most frequent or severe.

5—Phone use
4—Vocal strain (attempts to talk loudly)
3—Coughing

Voice Handicap Index

The Voice Handicap Index (VHI) scale, which seeks to assess the level of impact caused by the voice problem within three areas: physical, emotional, and functional, was rated by the client on a 0 to 4 severity scale (0 = never; 4 = always).
Total VHI score: 58/120
Subscale scores:
16/40 Physical
22/40 Functional
20/40 Emotional

Resonation

No hypernasality heard.

Articulation

No dysarthria noted.

VEGETATIVE LARYNGEAL FUNCTIONS

Tina's cough and throat clear evidenced moderate to good strength. She coughed frequently during the session, with increased coughing noted during effortful voice use.

TRIAL THERAPY

The following facilitative techniques were tried with no appreciable change in voice quality or loudness: falsetto voice, change in head positioning, Resonant Voice Therapy, singing. These techniques produced marginal improvement: using a cough, throat clear, or glottal attack to initiate phonation. Sustaining a /z/ "buzzing" sound was most effective in achieving a clearer vocal quality. Using a buzzing sound, Tina could sustain sound for 10 seconds and modify pitch in a controlled way.

SUMMARY

This 35-year-old female presents with vocal characteristics consistent with vocal fold paralysis with the exception of the sound of her cough and throat clear. She was diagnosed with iatrogenic left recurrent laryngeal nerve paralysis through laryngeal examination and CT scan. Before this evaluation, she was examined by a second otolaryngologist and reported to have full vocal fold movement bilaterally with a large posterior glottal chink. The client expresses confusion and frustration with her diagnosis and voice limitations. Diagnostic voice therapy is recommended. Based on the physician report, the moderately strong cough and throat clear, the variation in her phrasing depending on the speech task, and her success with trial therapy, it is hypothesized that her vocal fold has regained function but that she has retained the muscle tension voice patterns that she developed during the paralysis period.

RECOMMENDATIONS

The following recommendations were given to the client:
1. Participate in voice therapy to help determine an accurate voice and medical diagnosis.

Copyright © 2007 by Mosby, Inc., an affiliate of Elsevier Inc. All rights reserved.

2. Reduce vocal strain and improve vocal hygiene.

3. Undergo videostroboscopy to rule out a vocal fold motion impairment.

Long-term Goal

■ Tina will effectively communicate at home and at work through achieving her best voice possible through voice therapy as assessed through significant score improvement on the Voice Handicap Index, as well as improved ratings on the CAPE-V.

Short-term Goals

1. Tina will use Vocal Function Exercises and other voice facilitative techniques to improve the strength and functionality of her voice as assessed through pretreatment and posttreatment perceptual and acoustic measures.

2. The speech-language pathologist will be observant for a psychogenic or malingering component to this voice disorder.

POSTTREATMENT STATUS

After three voice therapy sessions with marginal progress, Tina was seen for videostroboscopy. To this point she continued to insist that her vocal fold was paralyzed. Videostroboscopy revealed normal vocal fold motion for both vocal folds. When adducting for phonation, the vocal folds were observed to have a stiff, bowed appearance, with reduced mucosal wave, and reduced amplitude. When Tina coughed, full closure was achieved. She observed her vocal folds on the monitor and saw that the left fold was no longer paralyzed, indicating her potential for achieving a normal voice. She seemed relieved but equally perplexed for an explanation for her poor voice. It was explained to her that she had habituated a tense muscle "set" in order to produce voice when her fold was paralyzed and that she had retained the muscle tension despite a fully functioning vocal fold.

After two additional voice therapy sessions using buzzing to initiate voice in conjunction with laryngeal massage and real-time feedback for pitch and loudness control Tina's "old voice" was restored.

Copyright © 2007 by Mosby, Inc., an affiliate of Elsevier Inc. All rights reserved.

TRANSGENDER VOICE: MALE TO FEMALE

For the male speaker desiring to be female, whether through sexual reassignment surgery or through nonsurgical means, voice, speech, verbal and nonverbal language will need to be changed. Some communication aspects such as adopting a more feminine vocabulary, changing posture and mannerisms, and so forth are more easily altered than voice-related changes. Voice presents a greater challenge based on the laryngeal anatomical differences between males and females. Males have larger thyroid cartilages with a more pronounced angle where the thyroid lamina join. They also have longer vocal folds with greater mass resulting in a lower habitual pitch, a downward shifted phonation range, and a lower-pitched cough, throat clear, and laugh. Refer to the keyboard diagram in the diagnostic section of the book where singing ranges for sopranos and altos (female ranges), and tenors and basses (male ranges) are displayed (see page 113).

Among the many differences in male and female communication, studies have shown that the pitch of one's voice is most salient in determining his or her sex.[74] The dilemma for the speech-language pathologist is assisting the client in finding and habituating a pitch that is not falsetto, not injurious to the vocal folds, and will not "crack." One that will minimally cause the listener to be uncertain of the gender of the speaker. If this is not possible, working on increasing pitch inflections and staying out of the lower part of the phonation range makes the voice sound less masculine. Making the vocal tone softer, breathier, and forward focused adds to the perception of a feminine voice.

Included in the diagnostic section of this book is a checklist that will allow the SLP to evaluate all aspects of the transgendered client's communication. The findings from this will guide the SLP and client in determining a treatment plan.

Providing therapy to a transgendered client can be challenging to the SLP from many perspectives. Based on this author's experience, establishing and expressing honesty throughout the therapy process is very important. It is important to know whether something said by the therapist is offensive to the client. Likewise it is important that the client not experience "The Emperor's New Clothes" scenario, whereby the client is led to develop a false perception regarding their vocal communication.

Lynn (the case study that follows), has been an interesting and challenging client. She is over six feet tall, and biologically has a low-pitched, robust speaking voice. Her goal is to be able to speak in a public setting without drawing the attention of those who hear her. In short, she wants her voice and speech to match her desired gender.

Copyright © 2007 by Mosby, Inc., an affiliate of Elsevier Inc. All rights reserved.

CASE STUDY 9-1

Gender Identity Disorder: Transgender (Male to Female) Voice

Voice clip #17

BACKGROUND AND REASONS FOR REFERRAL

Lynn is a 50-year-old sales associate currently in transition from male to female. She was seen for a voice, speech, and language assessment at this clinic upon referral from another speech-language pathologist.

HISTORY

Lynn has been dressing and appearing as a woman in public for several years. She has been taking Estradiol, an estrogen medication, and is hoping to have sexual reassignment surgery when finances allow. According to Lynn's case history, she feels that she was "born in the wrong body."

Lynn is taking several other medications not related to her transition for hypertension, elevated cholesterol, and hypothyroidism. Overall, she is in good health.

Lynn denies previous voice problems. She has not seen a speech-language pathologist while in transition. She has listened to an audiotape of a transgendered speaker and has attempted to model a similar communication style.

Extensive counseling has accompanied Lynn's transition. She described a lengthy history of depression preceding her decision to become a woman. Currently she states that she feels very isolated from her family. She has a friend in her workplace that has been supportive.

Lynn is self-conscious about the fact that her voice sounds masculine while her presentation and self-image are feminine. She wrote on her case history form, "I'd like my voice to match who I am."

OBSERVATIONS

Lynn presents as a conservatively dressed, tall individual. Her posture and head positioning are feminine appearing. She has a soft laugh. She gives the impression of being shy, seldom initiating speech. Despite dress, make-up, and well manicured nails, she continues to give the visual impression of a male.

EVALUATION
Laryngeal Examination

Stroboscopic examination of the larynx revealed bilateral vocal nodules at the anterior 1/3, posterior 2/3 juncture. Additional observations: An hourglass shaped glottic closure pattern; slightly reduced mucosal wave in the area of the lesions; increased glottic and supraglottic compression during phonation.

Pitch

Speaking fundamental frequency for /a/ measured 145 Hz. Habitual pitch when demonstrating the higher-pitched voice that she is targeting was estimated at 170 Hz. Pitch range extended from 99 to 237 Hz, approximately eight whole tones. CAPE-V results for pitch revealed a moderate to severe discrepancy between the client's pitch and intended gender. Reduced pitch inflections covering a narrow range were heard.

Quality

The relative average perturbation was found to be within normal limits at 0.24, indicating an absence of hoarseness. There was mild breathiness in her voice presumably used to make her voice sound less masculine.

Copyright © 2007 by Mosby, Inc., an affiliate of Elsevier Inc. All rights reserved.

Loudness

She had a mean intensity of 61 dB during conversational speech. She used reduced loudness intentionally, so as not to call attention to her voice. She was sometimes difficult to hear.

Respiration

Normal breathing patterns were observed.

Voice Handicap Index

The Voice Handicap Index (VHI) scale, which seeks to assess the level of impact caused by the voice problem within three areas: physical, emotional, and functional, was rated by the client on a 0 to 4 severity scale (0 = never; 4 = always).
Total VHI score: 48/120
Subscale scores:
12/40 Physical
13/40 Functional
23/40 Emotional
Her present voice does not appear to impact physical comfort or functionality. It is most limiting from an emotional perspective.

Resonation

Resonance lacks "forward focus."

Articulation

Tongue carriage appears more posterior in the oral cavity. Articulator contacts evidence increased force, more typical of male speech patterns.

NONVERBAL ASPECTS OF COMMUNICATION

Nonverbal aspects of Lynn's communication were observed informally. Feminine aspects of nonverbal communication were observed in posture, eye contact, and laughter. Nonverbal areas that continue to appear masculine included lack of verbal and visual affirmation such as head nodding and saying "uh huh," as well as hand and upper torso movement and gesturing.

LANGUAGE

Use of feminine adjectives, feeling statements, and "tag" questions were not readily apparent in the client's language sample.

SUMMARY

Lynn presents as a transgendered woman. She wants her voice and speech to sound feminine. The differences between male and female communication were discussed across a range of issues, specifically in the areas of pitch, loudness, duration, articulation, language structures, vocabulary, and nonverbal behaviors.

RECOMMENDATIONS

Lynn is motivated to make changes to her voice and communication style. It is recommended that Lynn receive 1-hour individual therapy sessions weekly as well as group sessions that meet twice each month.

Long-term Goal

- Lynn will have increased confidence when speaking to unfamiliar listeners, as assessed through a 10 point score improvement for the emotional statements on the Voice Handicap Index.

Copyright © 2007 by Mosby, Inc., an affiliate of Elsevier Inc. All rights reserved.

Short-term Goals

Lynn's speech will evidence feminine attributes through incorporating the following characteristics as assessed through pretreatment and posttreatment perceptual and acoustic measures:

1. Increased pitch and pitch inflections
2. Breathier, forward focus, voice quality
3. Incorporation of more feminine verbal and nonverbal language patterns
4. Lighter articulator contacts

Copyright © 2007 by Mosby, Inc., an affiliate of Elsevier Inc. All rights reserved.

The mode of communication that one chooses to use after surgical removal of the larynx (laryngectomy) is based on several factors: the anatomical and physiological changes postlaryngectomy, the presurgical and postsurgical cognitive, motor, and sensory abilities, psychosocial factors such as co-occurring dependencies, motivation, and support structure, the geographical area in which the person lives, and personal preference.

Currently two postlaryngectomy speech options (artificial larynx use and tracheoesophageal speech) are most popular.[15] An artificial larynx most commonly is a battery-driven device (electrolarynx) that provides an artificial sound source from which the speaker articulates. Tracheoesophageal (TE) voice restoration uses a prosthesis (which is not the sound source) in a surgically created site to allow pulmonary air to be channeled from the trachea to the esophagus where it is vibrated by the muscle segment at the opening of the esophagus (pharyngoesophageal [PE] segment) for sound production. The prosthesis functions to maintain the patency of the shunt, allowing air to enter the esophagus, while preventing food, liquids, and saliva from entering the trachea. The advantage created by the TE puncture procedure is that by using pulmonary air, many of the prosodic features of speech (rate, phrasing, and inflections), as well as conversational loudness level, approximate that of a laryngeal speaker. The quality and pitch of the voice, however, do not sound like that of a laryngeal speaker because the vibratory source is the PE segment rather than that of the vocal folds.

Both of the speech methods described thus far, when all conditions are ideal, allow the laryngectomized individual to communicate at a conversational speech level effectively soon after undergoing the laryngectomy. Very little speech therapy is required. There is ongoing maintenance and expense for both of these methods because of the ongoing need for supplies. Additionally, access to medical care is needed for TE puncture prosthesis management.

Prior to the refinement of the TE puncture surgical procedure, many laryngectomized persons attempted to learn esophageal speech, a third communication option, with varying levels of success. Esophageal speech requires the individual to "inject" air into the esophagus, through any of several methods, and then expel the air, whereby it is vibrated by the PE segment for speech production. This method of speech is most limited by the fact that only a small quantity of air can be injected for each speech attempt, allowing maximally 2 seconds of voice in which to articulate. Short phrase lengths, inadequate loudness, frequent air injection with concomitant negative habits, such as stoma noise and klunking, are ongoing sources of frustration. Speech is learned following a syllable, word, phrase hierarchy, necessitating multiple speech therapy sessions. Despite this description that probably sounds quite negative to the reader, the author has heard and worked with many excellent esophageal speakers. Once they have mastered this speech method, there are no further needs, although having a back-up electrolarynx is always recommended. During the time that the client is learning esophageal speech, he or she has an ongoing relationship with the clinic or medical center, which seems to boost morale and troubleshoot any secondary medical problems for the laryngectomized person.

The case study of Harold is included in this book for two reasons. First, despite Harold's opportunity to have a quicker communication solution by way of using an electrolarynx or having a TE puncture as a secondary procedure, he wanted to learn esophageal speech. He would have been a good candidate for a TE puncture based on all of the factors presented previously, yet he did not want an additional surgery, or "something else to deal with." Thus, honoring the patient's choice is important for the medical profession to consider. The second reason why this study

Copyright © 2007 by Mosby, Inc., an affiliate of Elsevier Inc. All rights reserved.

NOTES

was included was to illustrate that problem solving is a large part of teaching esophageal speech, and it is important that the speech-language pathologist persevere with the patient who desires to learn esophageal speech until relative certainty exists that this option is not a viable one for the client.

The second case study, Joseph, aquaints the reader with the evaluation, prosthesis fitting, trouble shooting, and instruction required for tracheoesophageal speech success. The emotional repurcussions of having cancer and losing one's voice are illustrated in this example as well.

Copyright © 2007 by Mosby, Inc., an affiliate of Elsevier Inc. All rights reserved.

CASE STUDY 10-1

Esophageal Voice

 Voice clip #18

BACKGROUND AND REASONS FOR REFERRAL

Harold, a 66-year-old retired teacher, was referred for an esophageal speech evaluation. He has had a total laryngectomy and wants to learn esophageal speech.

HISTORY

Harold had a total laryngectomy with a left radical neck dissection due to a cancerous tumor 6 months before this evaluation. His postoperative recovery was medically unremarkable. He did not have radiation therapy or chemotherapy. Harold was seen for electrolarynx and esophageal speech instruction at an outpatient facility 3 months after surgery. Both intraoral and neck-type electrolarynges were tried; however, Harold objected to the mechanical sound of these instruments and elected not to use either. He was educated about the TE puncture voice restoration procedure but expressed a lack of interest in having the procedure, indicating that he did not want to go through another surgery, nor did he want the maintenance of the prosthesis.

Approximately six sessions were devoted to esophageal speech instruction. Treatment was discontinued, however, due to a period of illness and lack of progress with esophageal speech. Harold was then referred to this clinic for additional input and instruction for the acquisition of esophageal speech.

The client describes himself as being in good health. He reports no major illnesses or chronic medical conditions. He eats all food consistencies. Occasional difficulty swallowing dry foods was reported. He does not have a hiatal hernia or any known problem affecting the structure or function of the esophagus. He has maintained his weight. He has good tongue movement bilaterally. Harold wears glasses. He denies hearing problems. He has discontinued smoking and alcohol use. No prescription medications are taken regularly.

Since his laryngectomy, he has noted belching associated with eating and also when drinking carbonated beverages. When he involuntarily belches, he can say words and phrases of two and three syllables. This was illustrated during this evaluation using soda. His esophageal voice, under this condition, showed no evidence of PE segment spasm or tightness. Harold has not been successful in belching voluntarily. He has not had an air insufflation test to evaluate the muscle tone of the PE segment.

Harold lives with his wife. He has two grown children. He enjoys reading and traveling. Presently, he communicates through "mouthing words," and writing.

ESOPHAGEAL SPEECH EVALUATION

Esophageal speech attempts were evaluated over two successive sessions.

Air Intake Method

The consonant injection and inhalation methods of air intake were described and demonstrated. Harold was not successful with either method. His attempts at consonant injection produced either a buccal or a pharyngeal sound, which were not consistent with the pitch and quality of voice heard when he belched with the aid of soda. All voiceless plosives, fricatives, and affricates were tried, without success.

When trying the inhalation method, Harold seemed to have difficulty following a motor sequence of commands. For example, he was instructed to keep his mouth open, while trying to "suck in air." He would close his mouth, even though he perceived it to be open. Using a mirror, and asking him to hold his mouth open with his hand did not help. Attempts at this method were discontinued.

Copyright © 2007 by Mosby, Inc., an affiliate of Elsevier Inc. All rights reserved.

Using the prephonation method of air injection, with labial closure, Harold was able to inject air into the esophagus as evidenced by the "klunk" sound as the air opened the PE segment. Clinician hand placement at the level of the PE segment gave further evidence that the air was entering the esophagus. During 38 attempts to insufflate the esophagus with this method, air was injected 20 times, yielding a 53% success rate.

Phonation

Although success was demonstrated with the prephonation air intake method, sound production after air injection was poor. During two speech sessions, only five volitional esophageal sounds (/a/) were produced. The average latency of the sound following successful air injection was consistently greater than 1 second. The duration of the sound of the five successful attempts was less than 1/2 of a second. Despite trying many techniques (i.e., verbal instruction; demonstration; altering body position and posture; using auditory and tactile feedback to time phonation onset), sound production was very challenging. From observing Harold's sequencing of air injection followed by phonation attempts, there was no obvious reason for his inability to reverse the air stream and phonate.

SUMMARY

This 66-year-old laryngectomized gentleman was seen for two diagnostic esophageal speech sessions. He is 6 months post total laryngectomy surgery. He reported minimal dysphagia, eating all food consistencies. The tumor did not involve the tongue or esophagus. He reported frequent involuntary belching but has experienced limited success with volitional attempts to produce esophageal sound. He presently writes and "mouths" speech to communicate. He is not interested in using an artificial larynx or undergoing voice restoration surgery. During the past two sessions, he has had success injecting air into the esophagus with the labial press prephonation injection method. However, he has not been able to reverse the injected air for consistent phonation. Based on his involuntary belching with resultant sound that has a pleasant quality and good duration, it is presumed that anatomically and physiologically he is capable of producing voice. It is hypothesized that esophageal speech is challenging because of difficulty in cognitively planning or motorically sequencing the process that produces sound. PE segment fatigue and a lax cardiac sphincter may be contributing factors as well.

RECOMMENDATIONS

1. To schedule the client for an air insufflation test to assess P-E segment muscle tone.
2. To pursue five trial esophageal speech sessions, after which time progress will be assessed and medical intervention explored, if indicated.
3. To practice the techniques introduced in therapy, for multiple, short, daily practice sessions.
4. To meet with and observe another esophageal speaker to aid in learning esophageal speech techniques.
5. To retry a neck type electrolarynx, to determine whether Harold's negative perception of it has changed.

Long-term Goal

- To develop esophageal speech that is functional and intelligible in all environments where background noise is minimal, as assessed by client and spouse report.

Short-term Goals

1. To volitionally and consistently inject air and produce voice with a short latency between insufflating the esophagus and producing voice.

Copyright © 2007 by Mosby, Inc., an affiliate of Elsevier Inc. All rights reserved.

2. To sustain phonation for minimally 2 seconds or for seven to nine syllables per air charge.

3. To reduce or eliminate all distracting visual and auditory behaviors accompanying speech production.

4. To establish and maintain intelligible speech through the coordination of phonation with articulation.

Copyright © 2007 by Mosby, Inc., an affiliate of Elsevier Inc. All rights reserved.

CASE STUDY 10-2
Tracheoesophageal Voice

BACKGROUND AND REASONS FOR REFERRAL

Joseph is a 71-year-old retired gentleman referred to speech-language pathology for alaryngeal voice and speech evaluation and treatment.

HISTORY

Joseph underwent four-vessel coronary artery bypass surgery after an acute myocardial infarction. One month after discharge, he presented to the emergency room with shortness of breath. The etiology of the dyspnea was determined to be respiratory rather than cardiac. Examination showed an obstructing laryngeal mass with bilateral vocal fold motion impairment. Joseph required an emergency tracheostomy to stabilize the airway. The lesion was staged as a T4, N0, M0 squamous cell carcinoma of the larynx.

This gentleman has a history of tobacco use but quit 5 years previously. He drinks minimal alcohol. Medical history is also significant for hypertension and borderline diabetes. He has not previously had radiation therapy.

The patient, after discussion with his family and physicians, elected to proceed with a total laryngectomy and primary tracheoesophageal (TE) puncture. He met with a speech-language pathologist for preoperative counseling. Joseph did not engage in discussion about postoperative changes and closed his eyes frequently during explanations. His family indicated understanding of the procedure, the expected postoperative changes, and postoperative voice and speech options.

The total laryngectomy was performed with a primary TE puncture, without complications. A videofluoroscopic swallowing study was performed on postoperative day 6, which showed no fistula. He was discharged home on a full liquid diet. During Joseph's hospitalization, a speech-language pathologist worked with him on electrolarynx use and continued to teach the patient about the changes caused by his surgery. He was discharged 7 days after surgery and was intelligible using his electrolarynx in known contexts with occasional need for repetition of words or phrases.

The outpatient tracheoesophageal voice and speech evaluation took place over two visits; 12 days after surgery and 24 days after surgery. The patient saw the otolaryngologist and clinic nurse on the same days. He was scheduled to begin postoperative radiation therapy in another 2 to 4 weeks.

TRACHEOESOPHAGEAL VOICE AND SPEECH EVALUATION
Diet

At the first evaluation, Joseph reported he was tolerating the liquid diet without difficulty. The otolaryngologist gave him clearance to advance to soft foods. At the second evaluation, he reported no difficulties with soft foods and was advanced to a full diet.

Stoma

At the first evaluation session, the stoma was patent and the sutures still in place. Joseph reported discomfort with light touch to the skin around the stoma. He was not wearing a stoma cover; the foam filters he received at discharge did not stick to his neck. His family asked questions about the functions of stoma covers and where to purchase them. Joseph did not show any interest in the discussion. At the second visit, the stoma was well-formed. It measured approximately 2 cm in length and 1.5 cm in width. The sutures had been removed. The stoma was clean, with minimal crusting. Joseph was wearing a cloth stoma cover.

Prosthesis Fitting

The otolaryngologist requested that speech-language pathology evaluate and place the prosthesis on postoperative day 12 and that voice production be deferred an

Copyright © 2007 by Mosby, Inc., an affiliate of Elsevier Inc. All rights reserved.

additional 2 weeks. At initial presentation, a 14 Fr (diameter) rubber catheter was in the puncture, maintaining the connection between the posterior stoma wall and anterior esophageal wall. The catheter was removed and a tapered dilator placed. The dilator was slowly advanced until the puncture reached 18 Fr in diameter. The dilator was removed and the puncture measured at 10 mm in length. A 10-mm 16 Fr InHealth indwelling voice prosthesis was placed using gel cap insertion. A 16 Fr (rather than a larger 20 Fr) diameter was selected because the patient's catheter was 14 Fr and he found the procedure uncomfortable. The patient also has borderline diabetes, which can lead to poor tissue health. It is thought that small diameter prostheses might be less likely than large diameters to cause breakdown of the tracheoesophageal wall when tissue health is marginal. The prosthesis was held in place for the gelatin capsule to dissolve, and then proper placement of the prosthesis was clinically confirmed. The prosthesis rotated easily in the tract, the valve lifted without resistance and reseated immediately. The patient produced voice when the speech-language pathologist occluded the puncture during an exhalation. There was no leakage through or around the prosthesis as the patient drank a glass of water.

At the second visit, the prosthesis was in place and the lumen was patent. The patient's wife reported cleaning it using the cleaning brush given to her. The tracheal retention collar of the prosthesis was grasped with a hemostat and there was a slight (approximately 2 mm) gap between the posterior tracheal wall and the prosthesis retention collar. The patient was able to produce voice when the SLP digitally occluded the stoma. There was no leakage through or around the prosthesis as the patient drank a glass of water.

Communication

The patient did not bring his electrolarynx to either visit, and he did not have a pen and paper available. He communicated by mouthing words, using gestures, and through facial expressions. At the first visit, he was encouraged to continue to practice the electrolarynx and instructions were reviewed. At the second visit, the patient was allowed to start using the TE puncture.

Initially, Joseph could not consistently occlude his stoma using either thumb; however, looking in a mirror helped him achieve complete occlusion. He demonstrated difficulty coordinating the voicing sequence (inhale, occlude, exhale and talk, remove finger to inhale). With practice, he achieved control over the voicing sequence. Speech was fluent. Articulation was precise. Resonance was within normal limits. The patient's wife and daughter understood his spontaneous speech.

At several points during the evaluation session, the patient and his family referred to emotional difficulty processing the surgery and the associated structural and functional changes.

SUMMARY

An initial TE prosthesis was placed and Joseph can produce intelligible speech using digital occlusion. He and his family demonstrated excellent technique for cleaning the prosthesis. This gentleman expressed feelings of depression today and his family echoed concern about his emotional well-being.

RECOMMENDATIONS

1. Joseph should practice talking and return in 4 weeks, when he next sees the otolaryngologist. At that time, the fit and function of the prosthesis will be reassessed, as will the quality and consistency of voice and speech production. The need for therapy and further education will be determined at that time.

2. Joseph is to call for reassessment sooner if any one of the following occurs: (1) the prosthesis begins to leak and he coughs when he drinks, (2) he has discomfort with the prosthesis, (3) he has difficulty talking, or (4) the prosthesis looks like it is falling into his airway.

Copyright © 2007 by Mosby, Inc., an affiliate of Elsevier Inc. All rights reserved.

3. If the prosthesis falls out or is pulled out, he should either place a catheter into the puncture and have his wife call the office or go to the emergency room.
4. Joseph will be referred to a psychiatrist for an evaluation for depression.

Long-term Goal

- Joseph will verbally communicate and be understood in all settings where background noise is manageable, through the use of tracheoesophageal speech and/or an electrolarynx.

Short-term Goals

1. Joseph will habituate the motor sequence needed for voice production via TE puncture.
2. Joseph will independently clean and care for the TE puncture prosthesis and verbalize the plan that should be undertaken if the prosthesis becomes dislodged or leaking of liquids is experienced.
3. Joseph will master correct neck placement, tone control, and articulation using his electrolarynx.

Copyright © 2007 by Mosby, Inc., an affiliate of Elsevier Inc. All rights reserved.

RESONANCE DISORDERS: ORAL-NASAL BALANCE

A discussion of the etiologies and treatments for resonance disorders is beyond the scope of this book. The case studies, the "Towne-Heuer Passage,"[31] the diagnostic page for detecting and differentiating hyponasality from hypernasality, and the resonance lab are included to assist the speech-language pathologist in hearing differences in resonance and knowing tasks to include in the diagnostic process. The term *nasality* is known by most lay and professional people alike, but is often used incorrectly to denote any deviance in voice or resonance. Thus when a referral is made with the chief complaint being "nasality," the speech-language pathologist should be prepared for anything!

Hypernasality is a term that denotes an imbalance of oral-nasal resonance caused by increased nasality. It is the result of increased air passing through the nasal cavity because of the position, structure, or function of the velum as it attempts to maintain contact with the pharynx. It varies in severity, often depending on its etiology. A spectrum of nasality might reveal mild nasality on one end, due to regionalisms, foreign languages, and mild structural and functional deviations. On the other end would be severe nasality, most likely caused by anatomical and/or physiological deviations resulting in significant velopharyngeal incompetence. Hypernasality is perceived as excessive nasal resonance on vowels and voiced consonants. When the incompetence disallows a build-up of intraoral pressure needed to produce plosives, fricatives, and affricates, the sound is emitted through the nose, which is called *nasal emission*.

An evaluation for hypernasal resonance should include minimally a variety of speech tasks focusing on voice, resonance, and articulation and an oral motor examination. Further assessment by the SLP (if the equipment is available) may include use of a nasometer (See-Scape®), which provides feedback regarding the presence of nasal air escape, or aerodynamic measures, which provide quantitative measures of air pressure and airflow from the oral and nasal cavities. The medical evaluation should include examination of the velopharyngeal mechanism while speaking, through use of an endoscope placed through the nose or through the mouth. When attached to a video camera, the examination can be recorded and reviewed for treatment planning. Radiographic studies provide information about the velopharyngeal mechanism through x-ray imaging.

The value of speech therapy differs depending on the etiology and severity of the problem, as well as on the surgical, medical, and prosthodontic interventions that are in place. The case study of Ashley in the "unsolved" portion of the book illustrates that even with a pharyngeal flap for cleft palate repair, voice, resonance, and articulation problems remain that require therapy. In cases of "functional" hypernasality, speech therapy often can remediate the problem. The SLP needs to be perceptive to those occasional clients who use a nasally emitted snort as a phonological process error most often substituted for sibilants that have otherwise normal resonance. This type of speech problem is correctable through therapy.

Hyponasality is the term that denotes reduced nasal resonance. It rarely has a functional cause, but more probably is caused by a structural deviation or abnormality such that airflow is decreased as it attempts to pass through the nasal cavity. The most common cause of hyponasality is due to enlarged adenoids that impede nasal air flow. A hyponasal speaker typically is very limited in breathing through the nose and may keep an open mouth posture for breathing purposes. Hyponasal resonance is most noticeable on nasal phonemes /n/, /m/, /ŋ/. The substitutions heard are [d/n], [b/m], and [g/ŋ] or a distortion of the target sound that is less nasal.

The SLP's role with the client with hyponasal speech is to accurately confirm that the resonance is hyponasal versus hypernasal, followed by a recommendation for

Copyright © 2007 by Mosby, Inc., an affiliate of Elsevier Inc. All rights reserved.

a medical examination of the oral, pharyngeal, and nasal cavities, best performed by an otolaryngologist. Treatment is based on the etiology for the hyponasality. In the case study of Allison, once her adenoids were removed, her resonance and articulation improved. She attended three speech therapy sessions after her surgery where the focus was on increased emphasis of nasal phonemes and improved articulator precision.

Occasionally, after adenoidectomy, the patient emerges with hypernasal resonance. Most likely adequate velopharyngeal closure was dependent on the presence of adenoid tissue, and once removed, the inadequacy of the velopharyngeal mechanism was revealed.

Copyright © 2007 by Mosby, Inc., an affiliate of Elsevier Inc. All rights reserved.

CASE STUDY 11-1

Hyponasal Resonance

 Voice clip #19

BACKGROUND AND REASONS FOR REFERRAL

Allison, a 14-year-old ninth grade student, was seen for a voice, resonance, and articulation assessment upon referral from a family friend who works as a speech pathologist. The presenting complaint was "poor enunciation and nasal speech." Her mother, who provided additional input, accompanied Allison.

HISTORY

Using a voice and speech self-assessment questionnaire, Allison identified these features as impeding her ability to be an effective speaker: a nasal sounding voice, sloppy articulation, and a fast speech rate. She feels that these speech characteristics have become more pronounced during her middle school years. According to Allison's mother, Allison is often asked to repeat her statements as a result of "mumbling."

Allison is in good overall health, free of allergies or frequent colds. She has not had her tonsils or adenoids removed. Her hearing is within normal limits. She has not had orthodontia treatment. She does not describe eating or swallowing difficulties and does not report nasal regurgitation of liquids. There is no visible sign of a repaired cleft lip or palate. She denies difficulty blowing up a balloon or talking loudly. Her birth and developmental history, as recalled by her mother, were unremarkable. She has had no previous speech therapy. Allison is a good student. She excels in both sports and the arts.

OBSERVATIONS

During the evaluation, Allison's resting oral posture was that of her lips and teeth being slightly parted and tongue slightly protruded. While quietly completing the self-assessment form, breathing through her nose seemed slightly effortful and was audible to the examiner. Throughout the evaluation Allison gave the impression of having a "stopped up nose," although she denied having a cold and said that breathing in this manner was normal for her. Her mother denied that Allison snores at night, but stated that she often sleeps with her mouth open.

RESONATION

A perceptual evaluation was conducted using many tasks to diagnose and discriminate hypernasality from hyponasality. Using high-pressure consonants in words, phrases, and rote speech designed to elicit hypernasality, no instances of excessive nasality, or nasal "snorting" were noted. Rather, resonance seemed to lack nasality. Inadequate oral-nasal balance was noted throughout all speech samples, with hyponasality greatest on /n/, /m/, and /ŋ/. In using contrasting oral–nasal word pairs (i.e., bag and bang, bake and make), inadequate nasal resonance occurred on 85% of the nasal sounds, with /ŋ/ being most hyponasal (pronounced as /g/) and interfering most with speech intelligibility. Allison was asked to count from 90 to 100 with a small mirror held below her nose. Very minimal fogging of the mirror was noted during the production of nasal consonants, suggesting reduced nasal airflow when speaking.

ARTICULATION

There were no phonemes consistently misarticulated. Intelligibility was reduced because of hyponasal resonance and rapid speech rate, the later interfering with overall articulation precision.

Copyright © 2007 by Mosby, Inc., an affiliate of Elsevier Inc. All rights reserved.

EVALUATION
Voice

Quality, pitch, and loudness were within normal limits.

Respiration

Normal abdominothoracic breathing was observed throughout the evaluation.

Rate

Speech rate varied depending on the task. Conversational speech was more rapid than reading rate. When an accelerated speech rate was used, articulation precision was reduced and pause time between words was decreased.

TRIAL THERAPY

Allison was asked to read a paragraph while "overarticulating" the sounds in each word and deliberately pausing at commas and periods within the paragraph. This resulted in slowed speech rate and improved overall articulation. Using the cue to try to lower her soft palate and force more air through her nose while humming and saying nasalized phonemes /m/, /n/, /ŋ/ revealed no improvement in resonance.

SUMMARY

Allison presents with hyponasal resonance, affecting the overall oral-nasal balance of her voice. Reduced nasality is most noticeable on the nasal consonants, affecting speech intelligibility in some nasal-vowel contexts. In addition, intermittently her articulation lacks precision, presumably because of an accelerated speech rate. Based on trial therapy, articulation precision and speech rate can be altered through speech therapy.

RECOMMENDATIONS

1. Reduced nasal resonance should be further evaluated by an otolaryngologist to determine whether a structural abnormality is present.
2. Speech rate and articulation precision should be targeted through speech therapy. Both Allison and her mother were in agreement with these recommendations.

POSTTREATMENT STATUS

Allison was evaluated by an otolaryngologist and had her adenoids removed 2 weeks after this evaluation. She participated in three therapy sessions, which focused on improved oral-nasal resonance balance, articulation precision, and reduced speech rate, with a positive treatment outcome.

Copyright © 2007 by Mosby, Inc., an affiliate of Elsevier Inc. All rights reserved.

CASE STUDY 11-2

Hypernasal Resonance

 Voice clip #20

BACKGROUND AND REASONS FOR REFERRAL

Rose, a 46-year-old female administrator, was self-referred to this clinic. She described her voice as "airy and nasal" and questioned whether her voice could be improved.

HISTORY

Rose has been hypernasal since birth. She recalls very little about her speech during childhood but remembers receiving speech therapy in elementary school. She is one of four siblings that are living, having had two siblings born with a cleft palate that died in infancy. Rose does not recall having medical evaluations regarding her speech disorder but was told that she had a "soft palate problem." As an adult, she has not had an evaluation by a cleft palate team. An audiological evaluation conducted 2 years ago revealed a mild to moderate loss covering all frequencies in her left ear; however, a hearing aid was not suggested. She does not recall having her adenoids removed as a child.

Rose denies swallowing problems. She states that prolonged talking is fatiguing for her. Over the past few years she has needed to speak publicly to groups varying in size and has gained confidence as a speaker through doing this. Talking on the phone is a large part of her job, where she is often asked whether she has just woken up or if she is ill.

The client expressed an interest in possible treatment options. Additionally, she wanted honest feedback regarding her speech and the impressions that the listener formed upon meeting her.

OBSERVATIONS

Rose presented as a thoughtful, introspective woman who had not had many opportunities to discuss her speech problems, and now wanted information and honest feedback. Physically, there was no evidence of a cleft lip repair. Her dentition and occlusion were within normal limits.

RESONATION

Overall resonance severity was rated as four (moderate to severe). Hypernasality was consistent throughout the evaluation. Nasal emission was heard most often on /s/, /p/, /f/, and /ʃ/ sounds, with intermittent nasal emission heard on other consonants as well.

ARTICULATION

Because of velopharyngeal insufficiency, articulation of sounds requiring increased intraoral pressure lacked precision. This was observed most often on /s/, /sh/, /ch/, and /f/ phonemes. Overall articulation and intelligibility were rated as good.

EVALUATION
Pitch

Habitual pitch (SFF) was estimated at 196 Hz. Pitch inflections were reduced, covering the range of 196-246 Hz (three whole tones). Tremor was present in her voice, more noticeable on sustained vowels.

Quality

Using a 5-point severity rating scale, roughness was rated as 2 (mild to moderate) and laryngeal strain was rated as 3 (moderate). Hard glottal attacks and glottal stops were frequently heard. Laryngeal strap muscles were pronounced when she spoke.

Copyright © 2007 by Mosby, Inc., an affiliate of Elsevier Inc. All rights reserved.

Loudness

Appropriate for the treatment room with no background noise. Mean intensity was 69 dB. Reduced loudness inflections were noted. When loudness was increased, vocal strain and nasality were more pronounced.

Respiration

Normal abdominothoracic breathing patterns were observed.

Voice Handicap Index

The Voice Handicap Index (VHI) scale, which seeks to assess the level of impact caused by the voice problem within three areas: physical, emotional, and functional, was rated by the client on a 0 to 4 severity scale (0 = never; 4 = always).

> Total VHI score: 52/120
> *Subscale scores:*
> 19/40 Physical
> 13/40 Functional
> 20/40 Emotional

The VHI indicates that Rose's voice overall is functional for communication purposes but has physical limitations and emotional ramifications.

ORAL EXAMINATION

Structures of the oral cavity were within normal limits. There was no evidence of a bifid uvula, or a submucous cleft. The velum elevated when sustaining /a/. Velopharyngeal closure could not be visualized.

TRIAL THERAPY

The client was instructed to open her mouth wider and overarticulate to determine whether an appreciable change could be achieved in oral-nasal resonance balance. There was no change. She was also instructed to pinch her nares while counting aloud. This resulted in increased oral resonance and reduced hypernasality.

SUMMARY

This 46-year-old female presents with hypernasality, nasal emission, reduced loudness, and vocal roughness and strain. The reason for this has not been determined but appears to be anatomical based on her voice history as well as family history. The mechanism for velopharyngeal (VP) closure was explained to the client. Likewise, the effect that VP inadequacy has on articulation and laryngeal valving was discussed.

Rose is compensating very well for her resonance disorder through her efforts at overarticulating and overphonating. Today, there was only one phrase that the client said that was misunderstood by the examiner because of resonance issues. Information was shared with the client regarding diagnostic medical procedures for further evaluating VP function, as well as the professions that would participate in the diagnostic process. Treatment options were also discussed, with further explanation given about VP prosthesis. Recommendations for maintaining good vocal hygiene were provided.

RECOMMENDATIONS

It was recommended that the client think about the things that she had learned in the course of the evaluation and then contact the clinic if she would like to proceed with further evaluation. Without medical or surgical intervention, it is felt that little improvement can be achieved through speech therapy alone.

Copyright © 2007 by Mosby, Inc., an affiliate of Elsevier Inc. All rights reserved.

EVALUATION

CLIENT INTERVIEW

The voice evaluation form that follows, although appropriate for all clinicians of all experience levels, was created especially with new voice clinicians in mind. It is very comprehensive, allowing the interviewer to choose from a range of questions from which a pattern of responses will emerge to aid in differential diagnosis of the voice problem. During the client interview, it is not necessary to ask the questions in the order that they are presented. Often the client's responses will lead naturally from one question to another without the clinician even needing to ask the question. Through a series of questions that cover voice use as well as medical, social, emotional, and professional areas, clinicians seek to determine the following:

1. Whether the client's medical diagnosis is consistent with his or her symptoms and responses.
2. All possible etiologies for the voice disorder, bearing in mind that multiple etiologies can exist. (Just as voice misuse can cause structural laryngeal changes, so can organic and neurological etiologies cause muscle tension dysphonias.)
3. Whether the client is an appropriate candidate for voice therapy based on the diagnosis and his or her attitude toward treatment.
4. Whether the expertise of other disciplines is needed to provide the highest level of client care.
5. How the information shared by the client at the initial evaluation session can be used to document treatment effectiveness.

Some specific question areas deserve further comment, for which additional diagnostic "tools" within this book will be helpful. Dysphonia caused by gastroesophageal reflux (GERD), also termed *laryngopharyngeal reflux (LPR)*, has gained increased recognition.[73] Thus it is important that the clinician be familiar with and sensitive toward the signs and symptoms of GERD. In addition to the symptoms provided in the medical history portion of the evaluation, the reflux symptom index (RSI),[12] created at the Center for Voice and Swallowing Disorders at Wake Forest University, is included in this book. If symptoms of LPR are present, the RSI should be administered, with a recommendation made for a medical referral depending on the RSI score.

The Voice Handicap Index,[36] is an excellent tool to aid clinicians in determining the impact the voice disorder has on the patient—physically, functionally, and emotionally. A rating scale composed of 30 items, which is included in this section of the book, when administered at the time of the evaluation and minimally again at the completion of therapy allows clinicians to assess the effectiveness of therapy and the client's level of satisfaction with his or her voice.

A vocal abuse rating scale is included on the evaluation form that allows clients (and their parents, if they are minors) to rate their voice abuse and misuse. It is often revealing to have the client rate these behaviors at the time of the evaluation and again at the first treatment session. Frequently their scores are increased at the first

Copyright © 2007 by Mosby, Inc., an affiliate of Elsevier Inc. All rights reserved.

session because their self-awareness of voice use has increased following the initial evaluation. This rating scale, when pertinent to the disorder and its etiology, can be used intermittently throughout the treatment program to evaluate progress and to establish subsequent goals.

It is very important that clinicians be cognizant of the emotional status of the client. The client's psychological health, which can be revealed through the voice itself, can be causing or contributing to the voice disorder. Listening intently to the client's message, in addition to the voice characteristics, and observing the whole person with regard to facial expression, posture, gestures, and nonverbal vocal behaviors can reveal much about the client. It is equally important that clinicians remember that the negative or anxious psychological state of a client can be created by the voice disorder itself (i.e., as a response to having a voice disorder). This is particularly true for professional users of voice, those with neurological voice disorders, and those who have "lost" their voice because of surgical removal of the vocal folds. Included in this book are a list of symptoms for depression[19,49] and anxiety.[48,58] Further assessment in this regard should be done by a psychiatrist, psychologist, or licensed counselor.

The SLP is encouraged to ask personal questions if it will truly assist the clinician in providing better care for the client. A simple test for clinicians to take before asking a sensitive question is that of first asking themselves, "Do I want to know this information for the client's gain or for my own personal interest?" Most consumers of health care currently have some level of familiarity with privacy practices of health care facilities. Patients typically sign a Health Insurance Portability and Accountability Act (HIPAA)[2] statement before receiving care for the first time at a given facility. None the less, clinicians still need to assure clients (and strictly adhere to it themselves) that confidential information will be used and disclosed only according to the HIPAA guidelines. Likewise, if notes are being taken, a recording is being made, or an observer is present during the interview or treatment session, obtaining client (or parent, if a minor) permission is a must if the goal is for the client to feel comfortable talking about sensitive issues.

EVALUATION TASKS

The evaluation tasks focus on the main components of voice—pitch, quality, loudness, respiration, resonation, prosody, and articulation. Under each category, tasks are listed to guide the clinician through the diagnostic process. Accurate perceptual—auditory, visual, and tactile—observations are of extreme importance for diagnosis and treatment planning. Although perceptual observations are subjective, they are the true means through which we judge normalcy. New clinicians (as well as the experienced ones) must always seek to sharpen their perceptual skills. It is for this reason that the case studies, both solved and unsolved, in this book include an audio voice sample as well as a written description of pertinent aspects of the voice in addition to client observations. A description of the Consensus Auditory Perceptual Evaluation of Voice (CAPE-V),[7,8] a perceptual evaluation instrument developed by ASHA Special Interest Division 3, is provided following the evaluation form. In addition, the "Rainbow Passage"[24] and the "Towne-Heuer Passage"[31] are included for encouraging standardization of tasks.

Acoustic and aerodynamic (objective) measurements add informative qualitative and quantitative input to the voice evaluation.[68,69] These aspects and measurements of voice are listed under each voice component. For example, pitch can be further analyzed to include average fundamental frequency, pitch sigma, phonation range, and frequency perturbation. It is recognized that many clinicians will have limited access to instrumentation and will rely on perceptual observations. Several voice tasks require only a watch with a second hand or a pitch pipe (or musical keyboard) and yet allow objective measures to be obtained. Refer to the list of materials and basic equipment required for the evaluation. Included in this section of the book are norms for varying voice tasks and a keyboard diagram with notes

Copyright © 2007 by Mosby, Inc., an affiliate of Elsevier Inc. All rights reserved.

(white and black keys) converted to Hertz. Making an audio, video, or digital recording of the client's voice during the evaluation tasks is of extreme importance for purposes of validating the clinician's observations, sharing findings with the client, and using the information for posttreatment comparisons.

A section is also included for assessing musculoskeletal tension (MST)[11,61,66] because this is so integral to diagnosing muscle tension dysphonia (MTD). The results of this assessment should be reviewed in conjunction with the client symptoms discussed in the medical history. Diagrams of the muscles of the neck[29] and larynx[11] are also included to aid the clinician in learning to visually observe and manually palpate the upper torso muscles that often contribute to MTD. The best way to learn, however, is to identify these muscles and spaces on people of different ages and body types. A referral to a physical therapist (ideally one who expresses an interest in learning about the larynx and voice disorders) is appropriate for the client who evidences dysphonia in conjunction with excessive MST.

Laryngeal visualization and imaging (especially stroboscopy) has gained increased popularity in the past 15 years within our field as SLPs have recognized its value. Based on Dr. Hirano's explanation of the layer structure of the vocal folds,[17,32] anatomical and physiological abnormalities (especially those associated with vocal fold vibration) can be diagnosed and treated with greater accuracy through stroboscopic imaging. When performed by a speech-language pathologist, it cannot replace the medical evaluation provided by a medical doctor nor can a medical diagnosis be made.[3] What it does provide, however, is a thorough analysis of vocal fold (and laryngeal) structure and, more importantly function, which allows the best treatment plan to be determined.

Included is a section to document laryngeal visualization and imaging information and findings for the clinician who is performing laryngeal examination or is part of a voice care team. The "Stroboscopy Evaluation Rating Form"[57] and the "Stroboscopic Assessment of Voice Form"[14] are included in this text. Many voice texts have detailed descriptions of laryngeal imaging rationale, methodology, analysis, and interpretation. Additionally, continuing education training classes are offered in many geographical locations to acquaint the speech-language pathologist with the knowledge and skills needed to interpret and perform laryngoscopy and stroboscopy. The purposes of vocal tract visualization and imaging and the knowledge and skills needed by the SLP performing it are discussed in several ASHA publications.[6]

Trial therapy should be part of every diagnostic session. When the clinician first begins to interact with the client, she should be listening for clues that indicate the potential for producing a better voice. Armed with multiple voice therapy techniques and knowledge of how each technique will alter laryngeal and vocal fold function, appropriate ones can be introduced briefly to determine the benefit of each. When clients hear, feel, or see positive changes at the outset of intervention, they are more apt to be compliant and have a positive attitude toward therapy.

The area of voice disorders requires a team management approach—of which speech-language pathology is an integral part. The valuable contributions of other professions must be continually recognized as we evaluate and treat voice patients so that appropriate and timely recommendations and referrals can be made. In addition to the medical field (otolaryngologists, neurologists, internists, pulmonologists, radiologists, gastroenterologists, etc.), appropriate recommendations and referrals include psychology (or others in the counseling profession), singing and voice instructors and coaches, physical and occupational therapists, dieticians, and other speech-language pathologists whose knowledge and skills in a particular area surpass our own.

Collecting and recording data, even though it may take up the majority of the diagnostic session or even require multiple sessions, is incomplete in and of itself in regard to solving the client's problem. The client comes to the appointment with minimally two basic questions: Is there a voice problem? Is therapy going to fix it? Answering those questions requires the voice clinician to review all of the information

Copyright © 2007 by Mosby, Inc., an affiliate of Elsevier Inc. All rights reserved.

NOTES

that the patient provided during the interview (that which was said and that which wasn't), the assessment (subjective perceptual as well as objective measurable data and clues), and trial therapy (what worked and what did not). Analyzing subjective and objective results, comparing them to the medical diagnosis, and filtering them through our knowledge base and our scope of "normal" are the final, most important steps in determining the answers to those two most basic client questions.

Copyright © 2007 by Mosby, Inc., an affiliate of Elsevier Inc. All rights reserved.

ASHA 2004 PREFERRED PRACTICE PATTERNS FOR THE PROFESSION OF SPEECH-LANGUAGE PATHOLOGY

#34 VOICE ASSESSMENT

Voice assessment is provided to evaluate vocal structure and function (strengths and weaknesses), including identification of impairments, associated activity and participation limitations, and context barriers and facilitators.

Assessment is conducted according to the *Fundamental Components and Guiding Principles.*

Individuals Who Provide the Service(s)

Voice assessments are conducted by appropriately credentialed and trained speech-language pathologists.

Expected Outcome(s)

Consistent with World Health Organization (WHO) framework, assessment is conducted to identify and describe—
- Underlying strength and deficits related to a voice disorder or a laryngeal disorder affecting respiration and communication performance.
- Effects of the voice disorder on the individual's activities (capacity and performance in everyday communication contexts) and participation.
- Contextual factors that serve as barriers to or facilitators of successful communication and participation for individuals with voice disorders or laryngeal disorders affecting respiration.

Assessment may result in the following:
- Diagnosis of a voice disorder or laryngeal disorder affecting respiration.
- Description of perceptual phonatory characteristics.
- Measurement of aspects of vocal function.
- Examination of phonatory behavior.
- Identification of a communication difference possibly co-occurring with a voice or laryngeal disorder.
- Prognosis for change (in the individual or relevant contexts).
- Recommendations for intervention and support.
- Identification of the effectiveness of intervention and supports.
- Referral for other assessments or services.

Clinical Indications

Voice assessment services are provided to individuals of all ages as needed, requested, or mandated or when other evidence suggests that individuals have voice or laryngeal disorders affecting body structure/function and/or activities/participation.

Assessment is prompted by referral, by the individual's medical status, or by failing a speech screening that is sensitive to cultural and linguistic diversity.

Clinical Process

All patients/clients with voice disorders are examined by a physician, preferably in a discipline appropriate to the presenting complaint. The physician's examination may occur before or after the voice evaluation by the speech-language pathologist.

Comprehensive assessments are sensitive to cultural and linguistic diversity and address the components within the WHO's *International Classification of Functioning, Disability, and Health* (2001) framework including body structures/functions, activities/participation, and contextual factors.

Assessment may be static (i.e., using procedures designed to describe functioning within relevant domains) or dynamic (i.e., using hypothesis testing procedures to

Copyright © 2007 by Mosby, Inc., an affiliate of Elsevier Inc. All rights reserved.

identify potentially successful intervention and support procedures) and includes the following:

- Review of auditory, visual, motor, and cognitive status.
- Relevant case history, including vocal use history, medical status, education, vocation, and cultural and linguistic backgrounds.
- Standardized and nonstandardized methods:
  - Perceptual aspects of vocal production/behavior
  - Acoustic parameters of vocal production/behavior
  - Physiological aspects of phonatory behavior
  - Patient's/client's ability to modify vocal behavior
  - Emotional/psychological status
  - Medical history and associated conditions
  - Observation or review of articulation, fluency, and language
  - Functional consequences of the voice disorder
  - Use of perceptual and/or instrumental measures, including—
  - Perceptual ratings
  - Acoustic analysis
  - Aerodynamic measures
  - Electroglottography
  - Imaging techniques such as endoscopy and stroboscopy (these procedures may be conducted and interpreted in collaboration with other professionals)
- Selection of standardized measures for voice assessment with consideration for documented ecological validity.
- Follow-up services to monitor voice status and ensure appropriate intervention and support for individuals with identified voice disorders.

Setting, Equipment Specifications, Safety and Health Precautions

SETTING: Assessment is conducted in a clinical or educational setting, or other natural environment conducive to eliciting a representative sample of the patient's/client's voice production. The goals of the assessment and the WHO framework are considered in selecting assessment settings. Identifying the influence of contextual factors on functioning (activity and participation) requires assessment data from multiple settings.

EQUIPMENT SPECIFICATIONS: All equipment is used and maintained in accordance with the manufacturer's specifications. Instrumental measures may be used to assess voice production and/or laryngeal function. Instrumental techniques ensure the validity of signal processing, analysis routines, and elimination of task or signal artifacts.

SAFETY AND HEALTH PRECAUTIONS: All services ensure the safety of the patient/client and clinician and adhere to universal health precautions (e.g., prevention of bodily injury and transmission of infectious disease).

Laryngeal imaging techniques and selection/placement of tracheoesophageal prostheses are conducted in settings that have access to emergency medical treatment, if needed.

Decontamination, cleaning, disinfection, and sterilization of multiple-use equipment before reuse are carried out according to facility-specific infection control policies and procedures and according to the manufacturer's instructions.

Documentation

Documentation includes pertinent background information, results and interpretation, prognosis, and recommendations. Recommendations may include the need for further assessment, follow-up, or referral. When treatment is recommended, information is provided concerning frequency, estimated duration, and type of service (e.g., individual, group, home program) required.

Copyright © 2007 by Mosby, Inc., an affiliate of Elsevier Inc. All rights reserved.

Documentation addresses the type and severity of the voice disorder or difference and associated conditions (e.g., medical diagnoses).

Documentation includes summaries of previous services in accordance with all relevant legal and agency guidelines.

The privacy and security of documentation are maintained in compliance with the regulations of the Health Insurance Portability and Accountability Act (HIPAA), Family Educational Rights and Privacy Act (FERPA), and other state and federal laws.

Results of the assessment are reported to the individual and family/caregivers, as appropriate.

Reports are distributed to the referral source and other professionals when appropriate and with written consent.

ASHA Policy Documents and Selected References

American Speech-Language-Hearing Association. (1993). Position statement and guidelines for oral and oropharyngeal prostheses. *ASHA, 35*(Suppl. 10), 14–16.

American Speech-Language-Hearing Association. (1993). Position statement and guidelines on the use of voice prostheses in tracheotomized persons with or without ventilatory dependence. *ASHA, 35*(Suppl. 10), 17–20.

American Speech-Language-Hearing Association. (1998). Roles of otolaryngologists and speech-language pathologists in the performance and interpretation of strobovideolaryngoscopy. *ASHA, 40*(Suppl. 18), 32.

American Speech-Language-Hearing Association. (2004). Knowledge and skills for speech-language pathologists with respect to evaluation and treatment for tracheoesophageal puncture and prosthesis. *ASHA Supplement 24*, 166–177.

American Speech-Language-Hearing Association. (2004). Knowledge and skills for speech-language pathologists with respect to vocal tract visualization and imaging. *ASHA Supplement 24*, 184–192.

American Speech-Language-Hearing Association. (2004). Roles and responsibilities of speech-language pathologists with respect to evaluation and treatment for tracheoesophageal puncture and prosthesis: Position statement. *ASHA Supplement 24*, 63.

American Speech-Language-Hearing Association. (2004). Roles and responsibilities of speech-language pathologists with respect to evaluation and treatment for tracheoesophageal puncture and prosthesis: Technical report. *ASHA Supplement 24*, 135–139.

American Speech-Language-Hearing Association. (2004). Vocal tract visualization and imaging: Position statement. *ASHA Supplement 24*, 64.

American Speech-Language-Hearing Association. (2004). Vocal tract visualization and imaging: Technical report. *ASHA Supplement 24*, 140–145.

World Health Organization. (2001). International classification of functioning, disability and health. Geneva, Switzerland: Author.

Reprinted from American Speech-Language-Hearing Association: *Preferred practice patterns for the profession of speech-language pathology*, 2004. Retrieved February 28, 2005, from http://www.asha.org/members/deskref-journal/deskref/default

Copyright © 2007 by Mosby, Inc., an affiliate of Elsevier Inc. All rights reserved.

BASIC VOICE EVALUATION EQUIPMENT AND MATERIALS

1. Audiotape or digital recorder with a handheld microphone (less expensive option: Fisher-Price, $40.00)
2. Cassette tape
3. Pitch pipe—if no computerized equipment is available (A 440 C4-C5 Music Store, $25.00)
4. Stopwatch or clock with a second hand
5. Voice evaluation form
6. Norms for pitch, duration, /s/:/z/ ratio, etc.
7. CAPE-V sentences and rating form[7,8]
8. Voice handicap index[36]
9. Standardized reading passage such as "Rainbow Passage"[24]
10. Tongue depressor
11. Flashlight
12. Gloves
13. Mirror
14. Water for the client
15. Tissues
16. Alcohol wipes to clean microphones
17. Picture or model of the larynx and vocal folds

Copyright © 2007 by Mosby, Inc., an affiliate of Elsevier Inc. All rights reserved.

TASK MODIFICATIONS AND PROPS FOR CHILDREN

1. To obtain a speech sample for nonreaders that can be repeated for posttherapy comparisons:

> *Count to 10 or 20; say ABCs; recite nursery rhymes (have book available); recite "Pledge of Allegiance."*

2. To elicit pitch range or teach the concept of high and low pitches:

> *Build Lego steps and have a figurine to accompany; use a picture or a model of a ladder, skyscraper, or Ferris wheel; have a small toy fire engine or ambulance; use a pretend cupcake and candle for singing "Happy Birthday."*

3. To elicit dynamic range or teach the concept of loud and quiet speech:

> *Use a puppet whose mouth can be opened minimally and maximally; use small and large stuffed bears to contrast the loudness of their growls; use a toy drum with a feather and a drumstick.*

4. To elicit S/Z ratio:[21,70]

> *Move a toy snake as the child hisses; use a plastic inflatable toy with a leak for /s/; use a toy car, motorcycle, or bumble bee to stimulate a buzz sound.*

5. To elicit a conversational sample use pictures and toy props:

> *Ask "how" type questions that involve a sequence; discuss birthdays, pets, and "boo boos" (requiring band aids).*

6. To rate and teach about vocal abuses:[52]

> *Use pictures from books, magazines, and advertisements that illustrate children engaging in these behaviors, or take digital pictures of the behaviors.*

7. To teach the concept of muscle tension associated with vocal effort:

> *Have child perform and contrast a motor task, such as writing his or her name, first holding the pencil tightly and bearing down hard on the paper, then repeating the action while releasing the tension.*

8. To teach blowing techniques for habit cough therapy:

> *Use pinwheels, large feathers, bubbles, kazoos, bottle with narrow opening.*

9. To assess and teach about excessive nasality:

> *Hold small mirror under nose and have client repeat non-nasal phonemes and words.*
>
> *Place feather or tissue paper strip directly under nose to show nasal air flow.*

Adapted from Champley E: The elicitation of vocal responses from preschool children, *Language, Speech, Hearing Services in Schools* 24:146-150, 1993.

Copyright © 2007 by Mosby, Inc., an affiliate of Elsevier Inc. All rights reserved.

NOTES

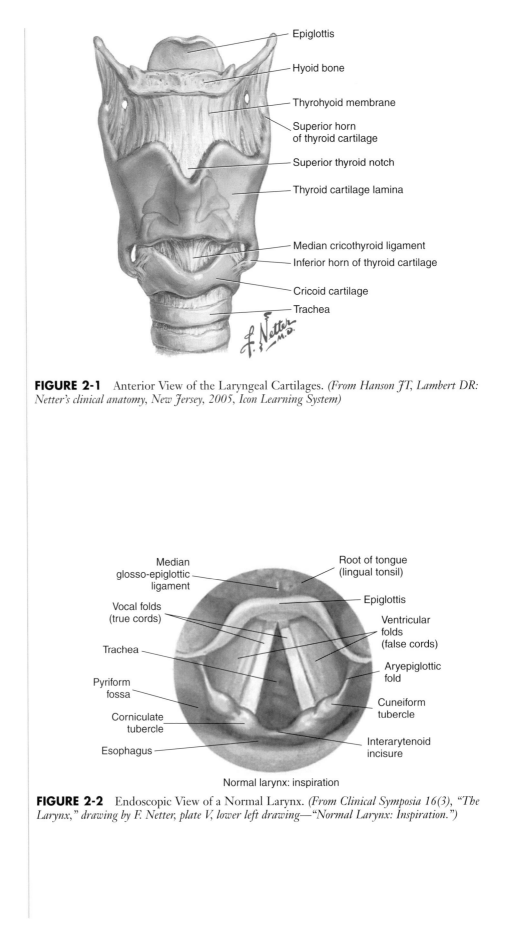

FIGURE 2-1 Anterior View of the Laryngeal Cartilages. *(From Hanson JT, Lambert DR: Netter's clinical anatomy, New Jersey, 2005, Icon Learning System)*

Normal larynx: inspiration

FIGURE 2-2 Endoscopic View of a Normal Larynx. *(From Clinical Symposia 16(3), "The Larynx," drawing by F. Netter, plate V, lower left drawing—"Normal Larynx: Inspiration.")*

Copyright © 2007 by Mosby, Inc., an affiliate of Elsevier Inc. All rights reserved.

SAMPLE OTOLARYNGOLOGY REPORT

HISTORY OF PRESENT ILLNESS

Today I saw Maddie, an 8-year-old female, for an otolaryngology consultation. She was referred by her pediatrician for evaluation of a hoarse voice. She has had progressive worsening of vocal quality during the past year. According to her mother, she yells and talks a lot. Her voice is worse at night and after she has used her voice loudly. It is also worse when she has postnasal discharge during the fall and spring, which is thought to be caused by allergic phenomenon. She does not have stridor or noisy breathing. She does not have exercise intolerance. She has never had surgery nor has she been hospitalized. She is otherwise healthy. She is in the third grade and doing well. She lives with mother and father and three siblings. There is no tobacco use in the household.

Medications

She is on no medications.

Allergies

She is not allergic to any medications. She does have environmental allergies at least symptomatically.

MAJOR FINDINGS

On my examination today, I found Maddie to be a healthy appearing young lady in no acute distress. She does have a hoarse, raspy voice. She is understandable, however. She has no stridor. Ears were examined and are normal. Nose is unremarkable. Pharynx is benign. Tonsils are moderate size. Neck is without adenopathy. Midline neck is normal.

She was scoped through the right side of the nose using a flexible scope. The supraglottic larynx is normal. Subglottis is normal. Vocal cords move normally. There is anterior to middle third junction fullness in each vocal cord, more discrete on the right than the left vocal cord. I suspect these are both vocal cord nodules. There is a remote chance that the one on the right may be a vocal cord cyst, but this is less likely because a cyst is much less common.

Plans

I have suggested consulting a speech-language pathologist with experience in voice therapy. If after 6 months of voice therapy she remains hoarse, microlaryngoscopy to definitely rule out a right vocal cord cyst is suggested. I would be glad to see her back if any problems arise. All questions posed by the family were answered.

Courtesy of Dr. David Tunkel, M.D., Associate Professor of Otolaryngology Head & Neck Surgery and Pediatrics Director of Pediatric Otolaryngology, Johns Hopkins Medical Institutions, Baltimore, Md.

Copyright © 2007 by Mosby, Inc., an affiliate of Elsevier Inc. All rights reserved.

ADULT CASE HISTORY

Name: _____   Date: _____

Address: _____   Zip: _____

Home Phone: _____   Cell: _____   Work: _____

E-mail: _____   Social Security No.: _____

Date of Birth: _____   Age: _____   Gender: _____

Place of Employment: _____

Occupation: _____

Referred By: _____

Medical Doctor: _____

Address: _____

Marital Status: _____   Name of Spouse: _____

Names and Ages of Children:

_____

_____

Person Responsible For Payment: _____

Insurance Company: _____

Policy Number: _____   Group Number: _____

Statement of present problem (be specific):

Describe previous speech/voice/language concerns.

Describe previous speech/voice therapy.

Surgeries (type and date):

Serious injuries (type and date):

Serious illnesses/Medical conditions:

Medications (include vitamins and herbal supplements):

Psychological/Counseling services (date):

Family history of speech/language/voice/hearing problems:

Date of last hearing test and results:

Copyright © 2007 by Mosby, Inc., an affiliate of Elsevier Inc. All rights reserved.

ADULT CASE HISTORY, *cont'd*

PLEASE CHECK IF YOU HAVE EVER HAD:

___AIDS	___Depression	___Indigestion	___Swallowing problem
___Allergies	___Diabetes	___Nasal blockage	___Throat clearing
___Anxiety disorder	___Dizziness	___Neck injury	___Throat dryness
___Arthritis	___Ear infections	___Neurological disease	___Throat pain
___Asthma	___Ear pain/ringing	___Obsession/compulsion	___Thyroid problem
___Bipolar disorder	___Eating disorder	___Postnasal drip	___TMJ
___Breathing problem	___Headaches	___Psychiatric disorder	___Tremor
___Cancer	___Hearing loss	___Seizures	___Ulcer
___Chronic fatigue	___Heart disease	___Sinus problems	___Weight loss
___Chronic cough	___Hiatal hernia	___Sleep problems	
___Choking	___Hoarseness	___Stroke	

Additional information that you would like to share:

Adapted from Rammage L, Morrison M, Nichol H, et al: *Management of the voice and its disorders,* ed 2, Vancouver, Canada, 2001, Singular.

Copyright © 2007 by Mosby, Inc., an affiliate of Elsevier Inc. All rights reserved.

CHILD CASE HISTORY

Name: _____   Date: _____

Address: _____   Zip: _____

Home Phone: _____   Cell: _____   Work: _____

E-mail: _____   Social Security No.: _____

Date of Birth: _____   Age: _____   Gender: _____

Grade: _____   Name of School: _____

Teacher: _____

Referred by: _____

Family Physician: _____

Address: _____

Person Responsible for Payment: _____

Insurance Company: _____

Policy Number: _____   Group Number: _____

Family e-mail: _____   Client's e-mail: _____

FAMILY INFORMATION

Father's Name: _____

Occupation: _____   Education: _____

Place of Employment: _____   Phone Number: _____

Living: _____   Deceased: _____   Disabilities: _____

Mother's Name: _____

Occupation: _____   Education: _____

Place of Employment: _____   Phone Number: _____

Living: _____   Deceased: _____   Disabilities: _____

OTHER CHILDREN BY AGE:

Name: _____   Gender: _____   Age: _____

Name: _____   Gender: _____   Age: _____

Name: _____   Gender: _____   Age: _____

CAUSE FOR CONCERN

_____

_____

DEVELOPMENTAL HISTORY

What maternal health problem(s) existed during the pregnancy with the child?

_____

General health of child at birth:

_____

Were developmental milestones met within the normal time range?

_____

SPEECH/LANGUAGE/HEARING

What speech/language problems did or do exist with client or other members of the family?

_____

Copyright © 2007 by Mosby, Inc., an affiliate of Elsevier Inc. All rights reserved.

CHILD CASE HISTORY, *cont'd*

Has your child been referred to a speech-language pathologist or had speech and language services? If yes, please explain:

Have you ever questioned your child's ability to hear?

_____

SCHOOL HISTORY

Child's attitude toward school:

_____

Is the child experiencing any learning or social problems in school? If yes, please explain:

_____

_____

_____

Area(s) of greatest academic interest:

_____

Area(s) of least academic interest:

_____

Is the child in an adapted program or receiving special services? If yes, please describe:

_____

SOCIAL DEVELOPMENT

Describe your child's social skills (e.g., is he/she independent, outgoing, cooperative, shy, neat, fearful, withdrawn, a leader, etc.)

What is his/her relationship with the following people?

Parents _____

Brothers/Sisters _____

Other adults _____   Other children _____

What unusual circumstances, *if any,* exist in the family?

_____

_____

HEALTH

Please describe the following in detail: medical or surgical treatment, any past or present illnesses or accidents, chronic health problems, history of medications, eating habits, sleep habits, history of allergies:

Has your child been seen for psychological or counseling services?   YES   NO

Is your child currently undergoing treatment? If yes, please describe:

_____

ADDITIONAL COMMENTS

Copyright © 2007 by Mosby, Inc., an affiliate of Elsevier Inc. All rights reserved.

TOURO COLLEGE LIBRARY

VOICE EVALUATION FORM

Patient's Name: _____ Date of Evaluation: _____

Medical Diagnosis: _____

Address: _____ Date of Birth: _____

Phone: (h) _____ (w) _____ E-mail: _____

Parent's Name (if minor): _____ Physician's Name: _____

Referral Source: _____

PATIENT INTERVIEW

(Assure patient of confidentiality; if taping, get signed permission.)

Voice History Interview

1. Describe your voice problem with as much detail as possible.

2. When did the problem begin?

3. Was the onset **gradual** or **sudden**?

4. What do you think is the cause of the problem?

5. Have you had previous voice or speech problems?   **Yes   No**

6. Have you had **voice evaluation** or **therapy** before?   **Yes   No**
    If yes, please discuss.

7. Has your voice **improved** or **worsened** since onset of problem? Have there been
    periods of normal voice?   **Yes   No**

8. Is the sound of your voice consistent throughout the day?   **Yes   No**

9. Under what conditions does your voice worsen or improve?

10. On a daily basis, how do you typically use your voice (occupation/type of voice use)?

11. How does your voice problem impact your professional or personal life?

12. Are there other family members who have had voice, speech, or hearing problems? **Yes   No**

13. Have you experienced increased worry, stress, or sadness preceding or accompanying your voice problem?
     (family, spouse, friends, work relationships, finances, health, school, employment)   **Yes   No**
     Please discuss.

14. Has your articulation (pronunciation of words) changed since the onset of your voice problem?   **Yes   No**

Copyright © 2007 by Mosby, Inc., an affiliate of Elsevier Inc. All rights reserved.

VOICE EVALUATION FORM, *cont'd*

15. Has there been any change in your mental (thinking, memory) abilities? **Yes No**

16. Has there been any change in your strength, movement, or sensation? **Yes No**

17. Has there been a change in your emotions? **Yes No**

PROFESSIONAL VOICE USE HISTORY (If applicable)

1. Describe how your voice is used professionally?

2. Have you had voice/singing training? If yes, are you currently working with a voice instructor/coach?

3. What are your professional voice-related goals?

MEDICAL HISTORY INTERVIEW

1. Laryngeal examination report—
   Name of M.D.: _____
   Date: _____
   Method: mirror, flexible nasoendoscopy, rigid laryngoscopy, stroboscopy
   Other findings:

2. How was your health at the onset of your voice problem?

3. How is your health today?

4. Have you had previous surgeries, trauma, accidents involving the head or neck, or chronic medical problems?

5. Do you have allergies, asthma, chronic sinusitis? If yes, how are these conditions treated?

6. Do you have symptoms of gastroesophageal reflux disease (GERD or LPR)?
   Belching _____ Heartburn _____ Nighttime coughing/choking _____
   Difficulty swallowing _____ "Lump" in throat (globus) _____
   Postnasal drip _____ Bitter taste in mouth (brash) _____ Habit throat clearing _____
   Symptom frequency: _____
   Symptom management: _____

7. Do you have swallowing problems? **Yes No**
   Describe.

8. Have you lost weight intentionally or unintentionally? **Yes No**
   If yes, amount of weight lost: _____

9. Do you have throat pain, irritation, or dryness?

Copyright © 2007 by Mosby, Inc., an affiliate of Elsevier Inc. All rights reserved.

VOICE EVALUATION FORM, *cont'd*

10. Do you have any of these symptoms of musculoskeletal tension?

    Headaches _____   Facial pain _____   Ear pain _____   Tinnitus _____

    TMJ pain _____   Bruxism _____   Numbness in hands _____   Shoulder and neck pain _____

11. Are you currently or have you previously been under the care of a mental health professional for diagnosis

    or treatment?   **Yes   No**

    If yes, please discuss.

12. Estimate your daily fluid intake.

13. Estimate your daily caffeinated fluid intake.

14. What medications are taken on a regular basis? (include vitamins and herbs)

15. Do you use tobacco?   **Yes   No**

    If yes, what type? With what frequency? Describe history of use.

16. Do you drink alcohol?   **Yes   No**

    If yes, what type? With what frequency? Describe history of use.

17. Describe the physical environment of your home and workplace. (air quality, space, noise level)

18. Is there any additional information that would help me better understand you or your voice problem?

VOICE EVALUATION

Voice Handicap Index

TOTAL SCORE: ___/120   **Physical:** ___/40   **Emotional:** ___/40   **Functional:** ___/40

Vocal Abuse Rating

0 = never; 1 = seldom; 2 = sometimes; 3 = often; 4 = very often; 5 = always

___Shouting/Screaming (+ or − emotion)

___Talking loudly (example: teaching)

___Excessive talking

___Talking in the presence of noise

___Phone use

___Singing

___Making noises/Imitating voices

___Forceful whispering

___Coughing/Throat clearing

Copyright © 2007 by Mosby, Inc., an affiliate of Elsevier Inc. All rights reserved.

VOICE EVALUATION FORM, *cont'd*

Pitch

Mean Fundamental Frequency

Sustained /a/ _____ Hz   **WNL?**   Yes   No

Mean Speaking Fundamental Frequency

Contextual speech _____ Hz   **WNL?**   Yes   No

Optimal Pitch

"Uh huh" _____ Hz   Sustained/ml _____ Hz   Laughter _____ Hz

Frequency Variability (Pitch Inflections)

Contextual speech _____ Hz – _____ Hz

Phonation Range

Musical notes (steps) Up _____ Hz   Down _____ Hz   **# of Notes** _____

Siren Up _____ Hz   Down _____ Hz   **# of Notes** _____

Highest from both tasks _____ Hz   Lowest from both tasks _____ Hz   **# of Notes** _____

Frequency Perturbation (jitter)

/a/ _____ %   **WNL?**   Yes   No

CAPE–V Pitch _____% too high or too low

Pitch breaks ___ Monopitch ___ Diplophonia ___

Quality

Perceptual Rating

0-5 scale or CAPE-V overall severity _____%

0 = normal; 1 = mild; 2 = mild-moderate; 3 = moderate; 4 = moderate-severe; 5 = severe

Roughness (consistent or inconsistent) _____ Breathiness _____ Aphonia _____

Glottal fry _____ Glottal attacks _____ Strain _____ Voice onset problems _____

Phonation breaks: Abducted _____ Adducted _____ Tremor _____ _____Hz

Noise: Harmonic ratio _____ *or* Signal: Noise ratio   **WNL?**   Yes   No

Glottal diadochokinesis (successive /i/ repetitions) _____ /second (norm, 4-6/sec)

Strength and sound of: Cough _____ Throat clear _____ Laugh _____

Endurance (speech/voice fatigue with prolonged counting) _____

Loudness

Average vocal intensity _____ dB SPL   **WNL?**   Yes   No

Dynamic range ___ – ___ dB SPL   **WNL?**   Yes   No

Amplitude perturbation (shimmer) _____ %   **WNL?**   Yes   No

CAPE-V Loudness _____ %   Too loud   Too quiet

Monoloudness _____   Loudness decay _____

Copyright © 2007 by Mosby, Inc., an affiliate of Elsevier Inc. All rights reserved.

VOICE EVALUATION FORM, *cont'd*

Respiration

Diaphragmatic/Abdominal ___ Upper thoracic (shallow) ___ Breath sounds ____

Maximum phonation duration /a/ ____sec ____sec   **WNL?**   Yes   No

S/Z Ratio /s/ ___sec ___sec /z/ ___sec ___sec Ratio___   **WNL?**   Yes   No

Mean number syllables/breath: Reading ___ Conversation ___   **WNL?**   Yes   No

Breath groups: Too long   Too short   WNL

Phonatory airflow: _____mL/sec /a/ ____ Hz ____ dB SPL

Phonatory air pressure: _____ cm/H_2O Successive /pi/ ____ Hz ____ dB SPL

Rate

Excessive _____   Slow _____   _____   **WNL?**   Yes   No

Words/minute: Reading _____   Monologue _____

Articulation

Diadochokinesis /pʌ/ ____ /tʌ/ ____ /kʌ/ ____ /pʌt ʌk ʌ/___ **WNL?**   Yes   No

Dysarthria: Yes No   Describe:

Consistent articulation errors _____

Resonance

Hypernasal ____   Hyponasal _____   Severity rating _____   **WNL?**   Yes   No

Horizontal focus: Front   Normal   Back

ORAL EXAMINATION

Significant findings   WNL? Yes No

MUSCULOSKELETAL TENSION ASSESSMENT (refer to muscle diagrams)

Visible strap muscles ____   Narrow thyrohyoid space ____   Tense TH space _____

Posture _____   Reduced mandibular range of motion _____

Reduced head range of motion: Side to side ____   Front to back ____

Muscle tightness: Sternocleidomastoid L R   Pectoralis L R   Deltoid L R

Splenius L R   Levator scapulae L R   Trapezius L R   Rhomboid L R

Suprahyoid muscles L R   Infrahyoid muscles L R   Tense larynx _____

Observations

Eye contact   Facial expression

Involuntary movement   Facial symmetry

Emotional status   Presence of scarring (head and neck)

Respiratory pattern and sounds

Copyright © 2007 by Mosby, Inc., an affiliate of Elsevier Inc. All rights reserved.

VOICE EVALUATION FORM, *cont'd*

Laryngeal Imaging Findings (attach form)

Flexible Nasoendoscopy _____   Rigid Endoscopy _____   Stroboscopy _____

Structure:

Function:

TRIAL THERAPY

Techniques Tried:

Results:

Perceptual:

Acoustic:

Aerodynamic:

Physiologic:

RECOMMENDATIONS

PROGNOSIS

TREATMENT GOALS

See references 12, 14, 36, 40, 53, 57, 61 for additional information to reference while administering this form.

Copyright © 2007 by Mosby, Inc., an affiliate of Elsevier Inc. All rights reserved.

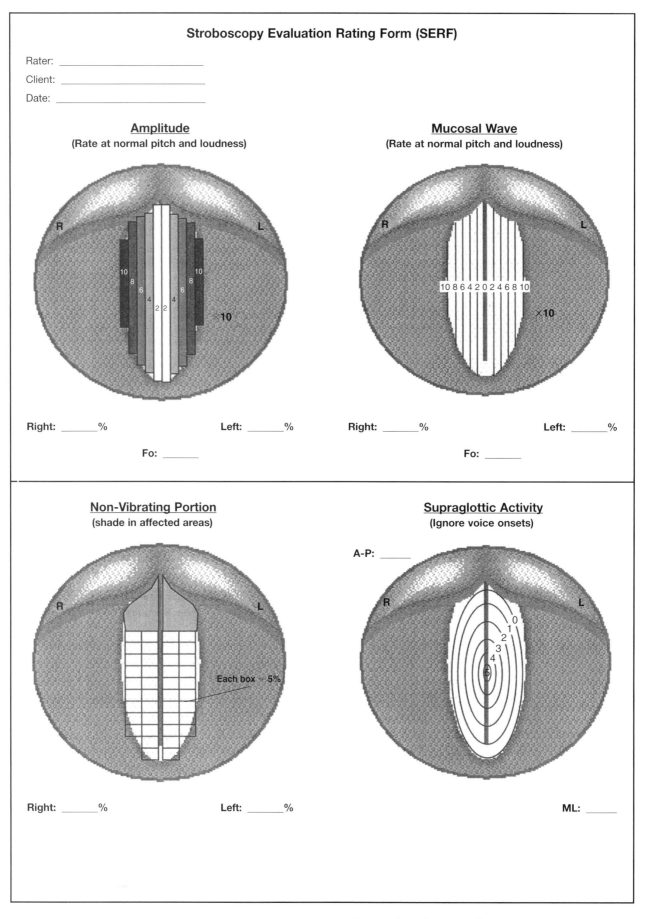

Stroboscopy Evaluation Rating Form (SERF)

Rater: _____

Client: _____

Date: _____

Amplitude
(Rate at normal pitch and loudness)

Right: _____%   Left: _____%

Fo: _____

Mucosal Wave
(Rate at normal pitch and loudness)

Right: _____%   Left: _____%

Fo: _____

Non-Vibrating Portion
(shade in affected areas)

Each box = 5%

Right: _____%   Left: _____%

Supraglottic Activity
(Ignore voice onsets)

A-P: _____

ML: _____

Copyright © 2007 by Mosby, Inc., an affiliate of Elsevier Inc. All rights reserved.

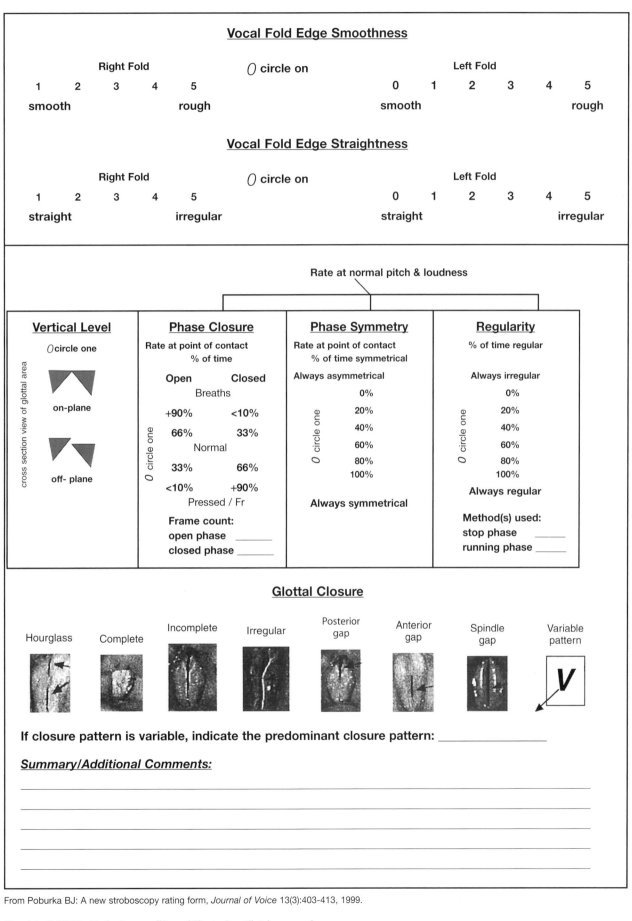

Vocal Fold Edge Smoothness

	Right Fold						*O* circle on		Left Fold			

Right Fold
1   2   3   4   5
smooth   rough

O circle on

Left Fold
0   1   2   3   4   5
smooth   rough

Vocal Fold Edge Straightness

Right Fold
1   2   3   4   5
straight   irregular

O circle on

Left Fold
0   1   2   3   4   5
straight   irregular

Rate at normal pitch & loudness

Vertical Level

O circle one

cross section view of glottal area

on-plane

off- plane

Phase Closure

Rate at point of contact
% of time

O circle one

	Open	Closed
Breaths		
	+90%	<10%
	66%	33%
Normal		
	33%	66%
	<10%	+90%
Pressed / Fr		

Frame count:
open phase _____
closed phase _____

Phase Symmetry

Rate at point of contact
% of time symmetrical

Always asymmetrical

O circle one

0%
20%
40%
60%
80%
100%

Always symmetrical

Regularity

% of time regular

Always irregular

O circle one

0%
20%
40%
60%
80%
100%

Always regular

Method(s) used:
stop phase _____
running phase _____

Glottal Closure

Hourglass   Complete   Incomplete   Irregular   Posterior gap   Anterior gap   Spindle gap   Variable pattern

V

If closure pattern is variable, indicate the predominant closure pattern: _____

Summary/Additional Comments:

_____
_____
_____
_____
_____

From Poburka BJ: A new stroboscopy rating form, *Journal of Voice* 13(3):403-413, 1999.

Copyright © 2007 by Mosby, Inc., an affiliate of Elsevier Inc. All rights reserved.

Videostroboscopic rating form providing an example of the relevant features to observe in clinical examinations completed preoperatively and postoperatively

University of Wisconsin VIDEOSTROBOSCOPIC RATINGS

Subject _____ Rater _____ Date of Sample _____

	Complete	Posterior	Irregular	Spindle	Anterior	Hourglass	Incomplete
GLOTTIC CLOSURE							

SUPRAGLOTTIC ACTIVITY		1 none	2	3	4	5	6	7 Ventricular phonation
VERTICAL LEVEL		1 glottic pane	2	3	4	5	6	7 off pane
VOCAL FOLD EDGE	right	1 straight/smooth	2	3	4	5	6	7 rough/regular
	left	1	2	3	4	5	6	7
AMPLITUDE	right	1 normal	2	3	4	5	6	7 reduced OR excessive
	left	1	2	3	4	5	6	7
MUCOSAL WAVE	right	1 normal	2	3	4	5	6	7 reduced OR excessive
	left	1	2	3	4	5	6	7
NON-VIBRATING PORTION	right	1 none	2	3	4	5	6	7 100%
	left	1	2	3	4	5	6	7
PHASE CLOSURE		1 normal	2	3	4	5	6	7 open OR closed
PHASE SYMMETRY		1 symmetrical	2	3	4	5	6	7 always asymmetrical
REGULARITY		1 regular	2	3	4	5	6	7 always irregular

Larynx (excluding folds) appeared: Normal   Abnormal

Vocal folds appeared: Normal   Abnormal

Epiglottis shape: Flat   Crescent   Omega

Mucous: Unremarkable   Remarkable

    — **Anterior mucous pooling**   — **Posterior pooling**

    — **Mucous ball formation**   — **Mucous stranding**

From Bless DM: Assessment of laryngeal function. In Ford CN, Bless DM, editors: *Phonosurgery: Assessment and surgical management of voice disorders,* New York, 1991, Raven Press.

Copyright © 2007 by Mosby, Inc., an affiliate of Elsevier Inc. All rights reserved.

CURRENT VOICE RESEARCH—ASHA DIVISION 3 – CAPE-V

One of the most significant research-based advances in the perceptual evaluation of voice has been the development of the Consensus Auditory-Perceptual Evaluation of Voice (CAPE-V) assessment tool. The CAPE-V is a perceptual voice rating instrument developed by The American Speech-Language Hearing Association's (ASHA) Division 3: Voice and Voice Disorders during a consensus meeting attended by clinicians, speech and voice scientists, and invited guest experts in human perception (e.g., visual, auditory, tactile). The meeting was held at the Department of Communication Science and Disorders, University of Pittsburgh in June 2002. After two days of presentations and discussion by clinicians, scientists, and invited experts, the working goal was to create a standardized instrument to rate perceptual attributes of voice quality. The tool would be suitable for judging all voice types perceptually and describing each according to a minimal set of salient vocal attributes—overall severity, roughness, breathiness, strain, pitch, loudness, and resonance. Additional goals focused on the expediency of administration and scoring, as well as versatility across clinical settings. The intended outcome for clinicians was to develop a consistent vocabulary and severity rating method such that voice disorders could be described and communicated among clinicians. The CAPE-V is not intended to be an exclusive measure of vocal function but to be used in conjunction with additional vocal function testing, including laryngeal imaging, to help create a composite set of data points for clinical study.

The procedure for the CAPE-V requires the client to initially sustain two vowel sounds. Next, the participant reads or repeats six sentences that have been carefully constructed to include various phonetically loaded contexts, including vowels /a, i, and u/, all voiced, oral plosives, nasals, /h/ onset, voiced onset, and other speech tasks that allow the clinician to assess the influence of phonetic demands on vocal quality. The final voice task is that of running speech allowing the clinician to perceptually evaluate the voice in a natural context.

A score sheet accompanies the CAPE-V. Scoring the CAPE-V is done using an unbounded 100 mm visual analog scale, where each perceptual voice feature is rated by placing a tic mark on the line. Guidelines are provided by the descriptors of mild, moderate, and severe below each line. The location of each tic mark when measured with a millimeter ruler provides a number based upon 100 mm, which corresponds to a percentage. Thus, an overall severity rating of 75 would fall in the "severely deviant range" with a score of 75% (75/100). Additionally the clinician determines whether each voice feature occurs consistently throughout each vocal task, or intermittently. Finally, blank 100 mm lines are provided for the clinician to list and rate other deviant aspects of the voice such as tremor, aphonic breaks, etc.

The CAPE-V emerged as the resultant procedure and documentation strategy from the consensus meeting. Although the CAPE-V has been actively used by clinicians in the field since 2002, the procedure and documenting forms have undergone several ratifying steps since its inception and has not yet been published in its final format by the field. Division 3 is currently conducting a national, multi-center field study to cross validate perceptual ratings using the CAPE-V with ratings made using the GRBAS audio perceptual scale. Participants will use both instruments to rate a large set of standardized voice samples, including both normal speakers and disordered voices. Findings from this research will allow Division 3 to finalize the CAPE-V format and procedures. For more information about the most current version of the CAPE-V procedures and score sheet, contact the Special Interest Division 3 program at ASHA.

Copyright © 2007 by Mosby, Inc., an affiliate of Elsevier Inc. All rights reserved.

Name: _____

Date: _____

Voice Rating Scale

	−			N			+
Breathing	1	2	3	4	5	6	7
(words per breath)	too few			normal			too many
	−			N			+
Loudness	1	2	3	4	5	6	7
	soft			normal			too loud
	−			N			+
Pitch	1	2	3	4	5	6	7
	low			normal			high
	−			N			+
Pitch Inflections	1	2	3	4	5	6	7
	none			normal			excessive
	−			N			+
Quality	1	2	3	4	5	6	7
	breathy			normal			harsh
	−			N			+
Horizontal Focus	1	2	3	4	5	6	7
	front			normal			back
	−			N			+
Vertical Focus	1	2	3	4	5	6	7
	throat			normal			nasal
	−			N			+
Nasal Resonance	1	2	3	4	5	6	7
	denasal			normal			hypernasal

Comments: _____
_____
_____
_____

The Voice and Voice Therapy 7th Ed, Boone D, McFarlane S, & Von Berg S. ISBN 0-205-41407-9.

Copyright © 2007 by Mosby, Inc., an affiliate of Elsevier Inc. All rights reserved.

RAINBOW PASSAGE

When the sunlight strikes raindrops in the air, they act like a prism and form a rainbow. The rainbow is a division of white light into many beautiful colors. These take the shape of a long, round arch, with its path high above, and its two ends apparently beyond the horizon. There is, according to legend, a boiling pot of gold at one end. People look, but no one ever finds it.

When a man looks for something beyond his reach, his friends say, he is looking for the pot of gold, at the end of the rainbow.

TOTAL WORDS: 100 (includes title)

*Compound word is counted as a single word.

TOTAL SYLLABLES: 129
SIGNIFICANT FINDINGS:

Client's Name: _____

Today's Date: _____

From Fairbanks G: *Voice and articulation drillbook,* ed 2, New York, 1960, Harper and Brothers.

Copyright © 2007 by Mosby, Inc., an affiliate of Elsevier Inc. All rights reserved.

TOWNE-HEUER PASSAGE

If I take a trip this August, I will probably go to Austria. Or I could go to Italy. All of the places of Europe are easy to get to by air, rail, ship or auto. Everybody I have talked to says he would like to go to Europe also.

Every year there are varieties of festivals or fairs at a lot of places. All sorts of activities, such as, foods to eat, sights to see, occur. Oh, I love to eat ices seated outdoors! The people of each area are reported to like us—the people of the U.S.A. It is said that that is true except for Paris.

Aid is easy to get because the officials are helpful. Aid is always available if trouble arises. It helps to have with you a list of offices or officials to call if you do require aid. If you are lost, you will always be helped to locate your route or hotel. The local police will assist you, if they are able to speak as you do. Otherwise, a phrase book is useful.

I have had to have help of this sort each trip abroad. However, it was always easy to locate. Happily, I hope, less help will be required this trip. Last trip every hotel was occupied. I had to ask everywhere for flats. Two earlier trips were hard because of heat or lack of heat at hotels.

On second thought, I may want to travel in autumn instead of in August. Many countries can be expensive in the summer months and much less so in autumn. November and December can make fine months for entertainment in many European countries. There may be concerts and musical events more often than during the summer. Milan, Rome, and Hamburg, not to mention Berlin, Vienna, and Madrid are most often mentioned for music.

Most of my friends and I wouldn't miss the chance to try the exciting, interesting, and appetizing menus at most continental restaurants. In many European countries food is inexpensive and interestingly prepared. Servings may be small but meals are taken more often so that there is no need to go hungry.

Maritime countries make many meals of seafood, such as mussels, clams, shrimp, flounder, and salmon or herring. Planning and making your own meals cannot be done even in most small, inexpensive hotels. One must eat in the dining room or in restaurants. Much fun can be had meeting the local natives during mealtimes. Many of them can tell you where to find amusing and interesting shops and sights not mentioned in tour manuals.

Reprinted with permission from Heuer R, Towne C, Hockstein N, et al: The Towne-Heuer reading passage—a reliable aid to the evaluation of voice, *J Voice* 14(2):236-239, 2000, with permission from The Voice Foundation.

Copyright © 2007 by Mosby, Inc., an affiliate of Elsevier Inc. All rights reserved.

MUSIC NOTES TO CORRESPONDING FREQUENCIES

- 8 whole steps = one octave
  A whole step is from one white
  key to the next white key.

- 12 semitones = one octave
  A semitone is from one white
  key to the next black key.

Lower ↑

Singing ranges

———	Bass	80-340 Hz
———	Tenor	95-550 Hz
———	Alto	140-700 Hz
———	Soprano	170-1040 Hz

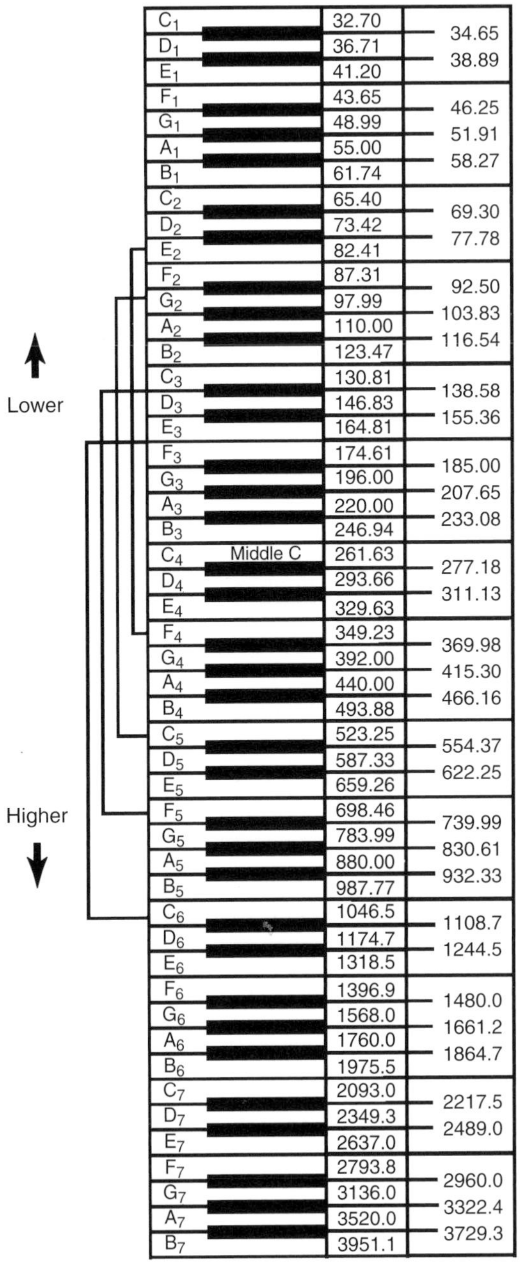

Higher ↓

Note		Freq.	Black key freq.
C_1		32.70	34.65
D_1		36.71	38.89
E_1		41.20	
F_1		43.65	46.25
G_1		48.99	51.91
A_1		55.00	58.27
B_1		61.74	
C_2		65.40	69.30
D_2		73.42	77.78
E_2		82.41	
F_2		87.31	92.50
G_2		97.99	103.83
A_2		110.00	116.54
B_2		123.47	
C_3		130.81	138.58
D_3		146.83	155.36
E_3		164.81	
F_3		174.61	185.00
G_3		196.00	207.65
A_3		220.00	233.08
B_3		246.94	
C_4	Middle C	261.63	277.18
D_4		293.66	311.13
E_4		329.63	
F_4		349.23	369.98
G_4		392.00	415.30
A_4		440.00	466.16
B_4		493.88	
C_5		523.25	554.37
D_5		587.33	622.25
E_5		659.26	
F_5		698.46	739.99
G_5		783.99	830.61
A_5		880.00	932.33
B_5		987.77	
C_6		1046.5	1108.7
D_6		1174.7	1244.5
E_6		1318.5	
F_6		1396.9	1480.0
G_6		1568.0	1661.2
A_6		1760.0	1864.7
B_6		1975.5	
C_7		2093.0	2217.5
D_7		2349.3	2489.0
E_7		2637.0	
F_7		2793.8	2960.0
G_7		3136.0	3322.4
A_7		3520.0	3729.3
B_7		3951.1	

FIGURE 2-3

Copyright © 2007 by Mosby, Inc., an affiliate of Elsevier Inc. All rights reserved.

A Compilation of Voice Norms for Phonation Duration, S/Z Ratio, Speech Rate, Loudness, Pitch

MAXIMUM PHONATION DURATION FOR /a/ (measured in seconds)

GROUP	AGES (YEARS)	MEAN (SEC)	SD*
Male young children	3-4	8.95	2.16
Male children	5-12	17.74	4.14
Male adults	13-65	25.89	7.41
Male seniors	65+	14.68	6.25
Female young children	3-4	7.5	1.80
Female children	5-12	14.97	3.87
Female adults	13-65	21.34	5.66
Female seniors	65+	13.55	5.70

From Colton R, Casper J: *Understanding voice problems*, ed 3, Baltimore, Md, 2006, Williams & Wilkins.
*Standard deviation.

S/Z RATIO
Calculated by averaging 3 trials of each sound, and dividing S/Z[17,21,70]

It is a measure of phonation efficiency when compared to respiratory efficiency. It does not diagnose the presence of laryngeal pathology.

- A quotient of 1.0 suggests normal vocal fold functioning.
- A quotient of 1.2 or greater in children suggests glottal valving inefficiency.
- A quotient of 1.4 or greater in adults suggests glottal valving inefficiency.
- Normative data for children through age 9 revealed longer /z/ than /s/ values.

SPEECH RATE—WORDS PER MINUTE

POPULATION	RANGE	POPULATION	RANGE
Children 6-8 years	119-130 words/min	Esophageal speakers	80-120 words/min
Adults (speaking)	160-170 words/min		
Adults (reading aloud)	140-185 words/min		

Data from Mathieson L: *The voice and its disorders*, ed 6, London, 2001, Whurr Publishers; Pindzola R: *A voice assessment protocol for children and adults*, Tulsa, 1987, Modern Education Corporation; Stemple J, Holcomb B: *Effective voice and articulation*, Columbus, 1988, Merrill Publishing; Wilson DK: *Voice problems of children*, Baltimore, 1987, Williams & Wilkins.

INTENSITY[9,17]

Average conversational loudness level is 70-80 dB (SPL)
Intensity range: 50 dB minimum; 110 dB maximum

From Andrews M: *Manual of voice treatment—pediatrics through geriatrics*, San Diego, 1995, Singular.

Copyright © 2007 by Mosby, Inc., an affiliate of Elsevier Inc. All rights reserved.

AVERAGE SPEAKING FUNDAMENTAL FREQUENCY[11,67]

Average adult female habitual pitch: 220-225 Hz*
Average adult male habitual pitch: 120-130 Hz*

*Standard deviation = ± 25 Hz

- Male and female habitual pitch levels are equally matched through approximately age 8.
- Voice (pitch) change for males and females usually is complete by age 15.
- After voice change, female habitual pitch has decreased by 2-3 semitones.
- After voice change, male habitual pitch has decreased by one octave (12 semitones).

PITCH RANGE
Range spanned from the lowest to highest frequencies[15]

Young, healthy adults: 2.5-3 octaves (20-24 whole tones).
This author (S.G.) has found clinically that adults with healthy voices who are not singers more typically have pitch ranges that span 16-20 whole tones.

Copyright © 2007 by Mosby, Inc., an affiliate of Elsevier Inc. All rights reserved.

LARYNGEAL AREAS MOST SENSITIVE TO MUSCLE TENSION

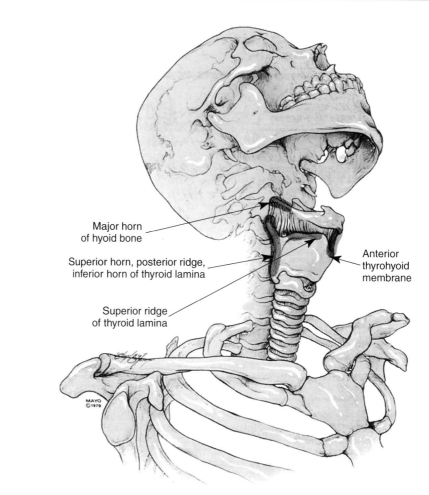

Major horn of hyoid bone

Superior horn, posterior ridge, inferior horn of thyroid lamina

Anterior thyrohyoid membrane

Superior ridge of thyroid lamina

FIGURE 2-4

By permission of Mayo Foundation for Medical Education and Research. All rights reserved.

Copyright © 2007 by Mosby, Inc., an affiliate of Elsevier Inc. All rights reserved.

NECK AND EXTRINSIC LARYNGEAL MUSCLES SENSITIVE TO TENSION

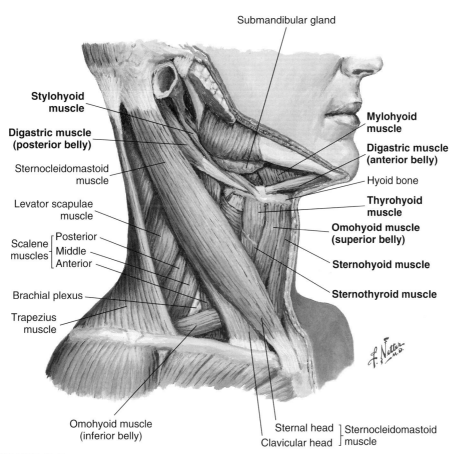

Submandibular gland

Stylohyoid muscle

Digastric muscle (posterior belly)

Sternocleidomastoid muscle

Levator scapulae muscle

Scalene muscles {Posterior / Middle / Anterior}

Brachial plexus

Trapezius muscle

Mylohyoid muscle

Digastric muscle (anterior belly)

Hyoid bone

Thyrohyoid muscle

Omohyoid muscle (superior belly)

Sternohyoid muscle

Sternothyroid muscle

Omohyoid muscle (inferior belly)

Sternal head] Sternocleidomastoid
Clavicular head] muscle

FIGURE 2-5

From Hanson JT, Lambert DR: *Netter's clinical anatomy*, New Jersey, 2005, Icon Learning System.

Copyright © 2007 by Mosby, Inc., an affiliate of Elsevier Inc. All rights reserved.

VOICE HANDICAP INDEX (VHI)

Instructions: These are statements that many people have used to describe their voices and the effects of their voices on their lives. Check the response that indicates how frequently you have the same experience.

(Never = 0 points; Almost Never = 1 point; Sometimes = 2 points; Almost Always = 3 points; Always = 4 points)

	NEVER	ALMOST NEVER	SOMETIMES	ALMOST ALWAYS	ALWAYS
F1. My voice makes it difficult for people to hear me.					
P2. I run out of air when I talk.					
F3. People have difficulty understanding me in a noisy room.					
P4. The sound of my voice varies throughout the day.					
F5. My family has difficulty hearing me when I call them throughout the house.					
F6. I use the phone less often than I would like.					
E7. I'm tense when talking with others because of my voice.					
F8. I tend to avoid groups of people because of my voice.					
E9. People seem irritated with my voice.					
P10. People ask, "What's wrong with your voice?"					
F11. I speak with friends, neighbors, or relatives less often because of my voice.					
F12. People ask me to repeat myself when speaking face-to-face.					
P13. My voice sounds creaky and dry.					
P14. I feel as though I have to strain to produce voice.					
E15. I find other people don't understand my voice problem.					
F16. My voice difficulties restrict my personal and social life.					
P17. The clarity of my voice is unpredictable.					
P18. I try to change my voice to sound different.					
F19. I feel left out of conversations because of my voice.					
P20. I use a great deal of effort to speak.					
P21. My voice is worse in the evening.					
F22. My voice problem causes me to lose income.					
E23. My voice problem upsets me.					
E24. I am less out-going because of my voice problem.					
E25. My voice makes me feel handicapped.					

Copyright © 2007 by Mosby, Inc., an affiliate of Elsevier Inc. All rights reserved.

VOICE HANDICAP INDEX (VHI), *cont'd*

	NEVER	ALMOST NEVER	SOMETIMES	ALMOST ALWAYS	ALWAYS
P26. My voice "gives out" on me in the middle of speaking.					
E27. I feel annoyed when people ask me to repeat.					
E28. I feel embarrassed when people ask me to repeat.					
E29. My voice makes me feel incompetent.					
E30. I'm ashamed of my voice problem.					

P Scale _____

F Scale _____

E Scale _____

TOTAL SCALE _____

Please circle the number that matches how you feel your voice is today.

Normal		Mild		Moderate		Severe
1	2	3	4	5	6	7

Reprinted with permission from Jacobson B: The voice handicap index (VHI): development and validation, *Am J Speech Lang Path* 6:66-70, 1997.

Copyright © 2007 by Mosby, Inc., an affiliate of Elsevier Inc. All rights reserved.

REFLUX SYMPTOM INDEX (RSI)

CENTER FOR VOICE AND SWALLOWING DISORDERS

WAKE FOREST UNIVERSITY

Name: _____

Today's Date: _____

Within the last month, how did the following problems affect you?

0 = No problem   5 = Severe problem

	0	1	2	3	4	5
1. Hoarseness or a problem with your voice	0	1	2	3	4	5
2. Clearing your throat	0	1	2	3	4	5
3. Excess throat mucous or postnasal drip	0	1	2	3	4	5
4. Difficulty swallowing food, liquids, or pills	0	1	2	3	4	5
5. Coughing after you ate or after lying down	0	1	2	3	4	5
6. Breathing difficulties or choking episodes	0	1	2	3	4	5
7. Troublesome or annoying cough	0	1	2	3	4	5
8. Sensations of something sticking in your throat or a lump in your throat	0	1	2	3	4	5
9. Heartburn, chest pain, indigestion, or stomach acid coming up	0	1	2	3	4	5
TOTAL SCORE*: (Sum of all columns)						

*The authors consider a score of 12 and below to be normal. (Personal communication with J. Koufman 1/25/05.)
Reprinted with permission from Belafsky PC, Postma GN, Koufman JA: Validity and reliability of the reflux symptom index (RSI), *Journal of Voice* 16(2): 274-277, 2002, with permission from The Voice Foundation.

Copyright © 2007 by Mosby, Inc., an affiliate of Elsevier Inc. All rights reserved.

THE STRUCTURES AND VALVES OF THE SPEECH MECHANISM

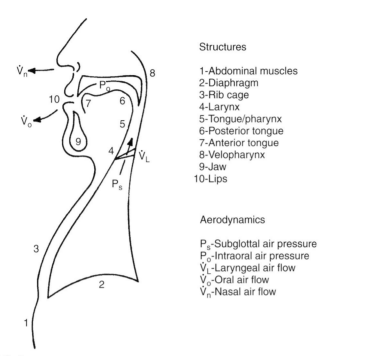

Structures

1-Abdominal muscles
2-Diaphragm
3-Rib cage
4-Larynx
5-Tongue/pharynx
6-Posterior tongue
7-Anterior tongue
8-Velopharynx
9-Jaw
10-Lips

Aerodynamics

P_s-Subglottal air pressure
P_o-Intraoral air pressure
$\dot{V}_L$-Laryngeal air flow
$\dot{V}_o$-Oral air flow
$\dot{V}_n$-Nasal air flow

FIGURE 2-6

Reprinted with permission from Netsell R, Boone D: Dysarthria in adults: physiologic approach to rehabilitation, *Arch Phys Med Rehab* 60:502-508, 1979. Copyright © The American College of Rehabilitation.

Copyright © 2007 by Mosby, Inc., an affiliate of Elsevier Inc. All rights reserved.

VAGUS NERVE DIAGRAM

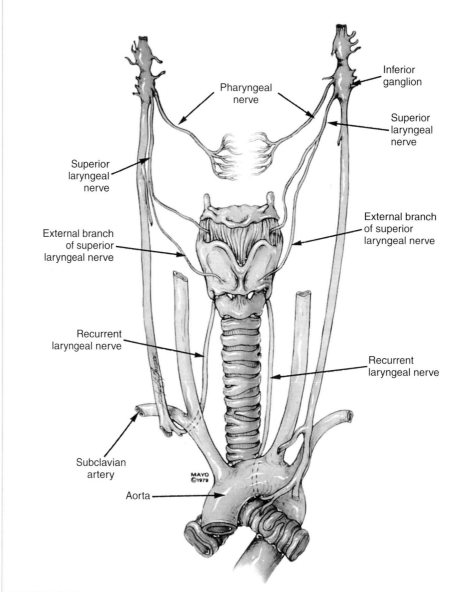

FIGURE 2-7

By permission of Mayo Foundation for Medical Education and Research. All rights reserved.

Copyright © 2007 by Mosby, Inc., an affiliate of Elsevier Inc. All rights reserved.

VOCAL CORD PARALYSIS

VAGUS NERVE INVOLVEMENT, LESION LOCATION AND EFFECTS—3 SCENARIOS

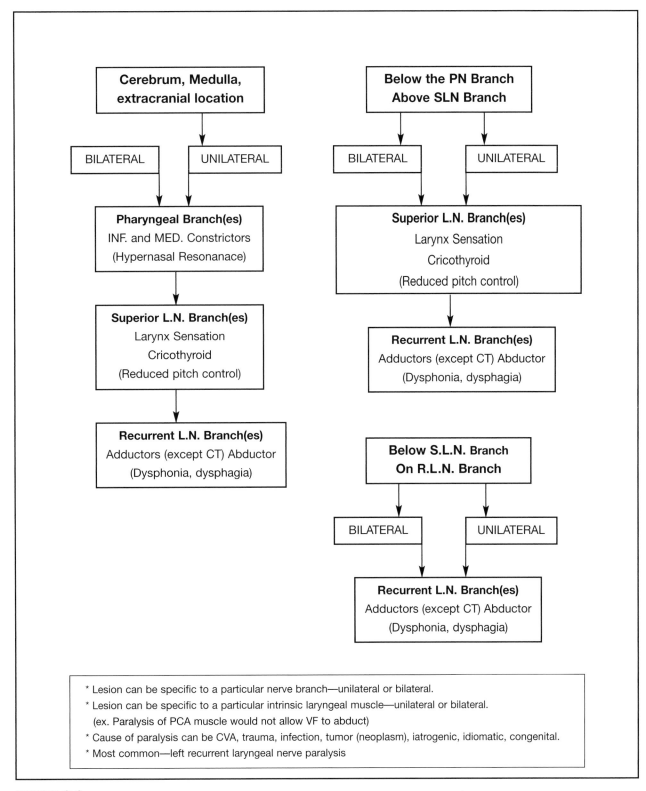

FIGURE 2-8 By permission of Mayo Foundation for Medical Education and Research. All rights reserved.

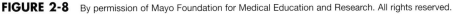

Copyright © 2007 by Mosby, Inc., an affiliate of Elsevier Inc. All rights reserved.

SPEECH AND VOICE TASKS FOR ASSESSING SPASMODIC DYSPHONIA

TASKS FOR ASSESSING ABDUCTOR SPASMODIC DYSPHONIA[22]

I. Sustained vowel /a/ several repetitions
II. Glottal diadochokinesis—successive /hi/ repetitions (4-6 per sec)
III. Connected speech (sentences and conversation)

> 1. *Potato soup tastes fine with crackers.*
>
> 2. *Patty, Casey, and Susie are sisters.*
>
> 3. *Cake and ice cream are tasty treats.*
>
> 4. *Tell Peter to paste his picture onto poster board.*

IV. Count from 60 through 80

Assess (perceptual and acoustic): voice onset time (prolongation of voiceless consonants); voice breaks; frequency shifts (pitch breaks); aperiodic segments (intermittent roughness); presence or absence of tremor.

TASKS FOR ASSESSING ADDUCTOR SPASMODIC DYSPHONIA[65]

I. Sustained vowel /a/—several repetitions
II. Glottal diadochokinesis—successive /i/ (4-6 per sec)
III. Connected speech (sentences and conversation)

> 1. *Ada and Eva ate oysters at the oyster bar.*
>
> 2. *All the girls made money by doing odd jobs.*
>
> 3. *Other than eels, Al likes all ocean animals.*
>
> 4. *Above the garage was an old, dirty, metal door.*
>
> 5. *Eighty, eighty-eight, eighty-nine, and ninety-nine were the winning numbers.*

IV. Read "Towne-Heuer Passage"
V. Singing, laughing

Assess (perceptual and acoustic): voice breaks (heard more frequently in vowels); aperiodic segments; frequency shifts (i.e., pitch breaks); length of time required to read passage or sentences; presence or absence of tremor.

Copyright © 2007 by Mosby, Inc., an affiliate of Elsevier Inc. All rights reserved.

SAMPLE OTOLARYNGOLOGY REPORT FOR SPASMODIC DYSPHONIA

HISTORY

The patient, Emma, presents for an evaluation of spasmodic voicing problem. She has a 14-month history of voice problems that have gradually worsened. She describes her greatest difficulty as speaking in a noisy environment and on the telephone. She states that she has more problems with one syllable words and producing certain consonants. She is currently on Prilosec (20 mg) per day.

EXAMINATION

On general physical examination, the patient is a pleasant young adult female in no acute distress. Her voice quality is abnormal, being low in pitch and markedly pressed in character. Regular episodes of difficulty with the initiation of speech could be heard that varied from hyperadduction to abducted breaks after voiceless consonants. No inspiratory stridor is heard. Regular episodes of throat clearing are heard. On palpation, the suspensory muscles of the larynx are tense but not tender. Her laryngeal crepitance was moderately to markedly diminished.

VIDEOSTROBOSCOPY
Procedure

Given the need to evaluate this patient's laryngeal function with running speech, videostroboscopy was performed using a fiberoptic nasolaryngoscope. The patient was asked to perform various laryngeal gestures, produce nonsense syllables, and read from a standard spasmodic dysphonia text.

Findings

The client's larynx is abnormal for the presence of mild posterior laryngeal edema and erythema. Her vocal folds are mildly polypoid with increased vascular prominence along the full length. Her epithelial wave is within normal limits. Thick mucus was stranding between the two folds. No evidence of recent hemorrhage or subepithelial masses could be detected. Both vocal folds are fully mobile.

When instructed to read the adductor spasmodic dysphonia passage, the patient demonstrated numerous episodes of difficulty with voicing onset and a tendency to hyperadduct her vocal folds and occasionally her false folds.

When reading the abductor spasmodic dysphonia passage, the client demonstrated numerous episodes of difficulty adducting her vocal folds, particularly after voiceless consonants. She did not appear to have any myoclonus or tremor-based component to her dysphonia.

IMPRESSION AND PLAN

The patient appears to have a combined adductor and abductor form of spasmodic dysphonia. It is recommended that she consider having her adductor dysphonia treated first with Botox injections to determine what benefit she will experience to her overall communication capacity. In the event that this only minimally improves her voice problem, we will proceed at a relatively short interval with a posterior injection to treat the abductor component. Furthermore, it is recommended that she start a regular dose of Prilosec at 40 mg/day to treat a source of chronic irritation that may be contributing to her tendency toward a MTD.

Courtesy of Paul F. Castellanos, M.D., Laryngology Bronchoesophagology, Associate Professor of Surgery, Division of Otolaryngology Head and Neck Surgery, University of Alabama at Birmingham.

Copyright © 2007 by Mosby, Inc., an affiliate of Elsevier Inc. All rights reserved.

NOTES

SPEECH AND VOICE TASKS FOR ASSESSING RESONANCE

PHONEMES for detecting excessive nasality[15]

VOWELS in isolation and in combination with nasal consonants
CONSONANTS requiring increased build-up of intraoral pressure may trigger nasal emission and nasal snorting

/s/ and /s/ blends	/f/ and /f/ blends	/tʃ/ "ch"
/t/ and /t/ blends	/k/ and /k/ blends	/ʃ/ "sh"
/p/ and /p/ blends		

SENTENCES without nasal consonants

1. Let's buy a big dog.
2. It's easy to tell us apart.
3. Four hours of hard work faced us.
4. Her purse was full of tissues.
5. Start the car please.

SERIAL COUNTING from 60 to 70

PHONEMES for detecting hypo (de) nasality

Nasal phonemes   /m/ /n/ /ŋ/

COMMON DE-NASALIZED SUBSTITUTIONS

/n/ resembles /d/

sample contrast words: **nose/doze and/add knee/Dee**

/m/ resembles /b/

sample contrast words: **mad/bad come/cub meet/beet**

/ŋ/ resembles /-g/

sample contrast words: **bowling/bow leg ringing/rig egg**

SENTENCES containing nasal sounds

1. Mom may know my meaning.
2. I know a man on the moon.
3. Nine young men owe money.
4. When may we know your name?
5. I'm naming one man among many.

SERIAL COUNTING from 90 to 100

Copyright © 2007 by Mosby, Inc., an affiliate of Elsevier Inc. All rights reserved.

Client: _____   Score_____/44

Date: _____

MALE-TO-FEMALE (MTF) TRANSGENDER COMMUNICATION ASSESSMENT

0	1	2
No	Some	Yes

Voice (Pitch/Loudness/Quality)

_____ 1. Habitual pitch is "gender uncertain" whereby the listener is not sure of the speaker's gender.

_____ 2. Natural sounding pitch inflections are used.

_____ 3. Overall (habitual) loudness is reduced.

_____ 4. Breathier (lighter) quality is used.

Prosody

_____ 5. Speech is fluid and melodious rather than choppy.

_____ 6. The duration of vowels are lengthened.

Resonation

_____ 7. A "forward-focused" (head) resonance is used rather than a chest sound.

Articulation

_____ 8. Increased articulation precision is used for all phonemes.

_____ 9. Wider mouth opening is used when speaking.

Language Vocabulary

_____ 10. There are more adjectives and adverbs used in conversation.

_____ 11. Descriptors used are feminine rather than masculine.

_____ 12. Less swearing, slang, and inappropriate language is used.

Language Structure

_____ 13. Indirect questions and tag questions and clauses are used.

Examples:

"Do you feel like eating something?" instead of "I'm hungry."

"I understand that—I think" instead of "I understand that."

"I'm not sure about those shoes, what do you think?"

Pragmatics

_____ 14. Communication is open and supportive, with nurturing phrases used.

_____ 15. Verbal and nonverbal supportive listening and understanding sounds ("uh huh") and gestures (head nodding) are used.

Body Language

_____ 16. Increased eye contact is maintained with conversational partners.

_____ 17. More facial expression and smiling are used.

_____ 18. Head movement is increased (side to side; head tilt; head nodding).

_____ 19. The speaker leans "in" or forward when speaking.

_____ 20. The speaker maintains more of a closed posture (contained, smaller movements) versus an open posture when sitting and standing.

_____ 21. More self-referential touching is used, such as playing with one's hair.

Physical Appearance and Fashion

_____ 22. Dress, make-up, scent is consistent with the image that the client desires.

Total possible score is 44 points.

Copyright © 2007 by Mosby, Inc., an affiliate of Elsevier Inc. All rights reserved.

SAMPLE PULMONOLOGY REPORT FOR VOCAL CORD DYSFUNCTION

HISTORY OF PRESENT ILLNESS

Today I saw Katie, a delightful 16-year-old who is a competitive swimmer, for a consultation. Over the past year she has developed shortness of breath with exercise. Her symptoms occur fairly reproducibly and only occur when she is swimming at high levels. She describes tightness specifically in her throat and intermittent stridor. It is harder for her to inspire rather than expire. When she stops for less than a minute, her symptoms resolve. She does not cough during the episodes. There are no palpitations or dizziness. Of note is that she has been on Maxair for the past year and uses up to 10 puffs in the course of a swim practice. It is unclear whether this has made any significant difference in her symptoms. She also has been treated with Flovent for the past few months without any significant change. Her growth has been normal. She experiences no overt reflux symptoms. Birth history and environmental history are unremarkable. Family history is significant for asthma in distant relatives. She has slight seasonal allergy issues and uses Zyrtec occasionally.

PHYSICAL EXAMINATION

Respiratory rate 16 and unlabored; weight 158 pounds; height 66 inches. Examination of ears, nose, and throat is remarkable for mild nasal congestion. Lungs are normal. Heart shows a normal rhythm without murmurs. Abdomen is soft; bowel sounds are normal and active, with no masses or tenderness. Skin examination is normal.

Labs Today

Oxygen saturation on room air was 99%. Spirometry measurements: forced vital capacity (FVC) 104% of predicted, forced expiratory volume in 1 sec (FEV_1) 106% of predicted, forced expiratory flow (FEF) 25-75, 98% of predicted. These results are all normal.

Exercise Challenge

Katie exercised on the treadmill well for about 13 minutes. During the last few minutes, she complained of fatigue and shortness of breath requiring the test to be discontinued. There was no desaturation during exercise. Her pulmonary functions before exercise were normal. After exercise, there was clear-cut flattening of the inspiratory limb of the flow volume loop consistent with upper airway obstruction. There was no change with bronchodilator. Within 10 minutes after exercise, her flow volume loop returned to normal.

IMPRESSION/PLAN

Katie's symptoms are directly related to the upper airway. I feel that she has classic vocal cord dysfunction (VCD) triggered by exercise. I do not feel that she has asthma. At this point, I recommend discontinuing Flovent and Maxair. I am referring her to a speech pathologist that is skilled in treating athletes with VCD. Both Katie and her mother were comfortable with this plan.

Courtesy of Dr. Samuel Rosenberg, M.D., Pediatric Pulmonologist, Pediatric Pulmonary and Asthma Center, Rockville, Md.

Copyright © 2007 by Mosby, Inc., an affiliate of Elsevier Inc. All rights reserved.

VOCAL CORD DYSFUNCTION

PATIENT INTERVIEW

Patient: _____   Date of Eval.: _____

Address: _____   Date of Birth: _____

_____   Occupation: _____

Phone: _____   E-mail Address: _____

Parents (if minor): _____   Referring M.D.: _____

I. DESCRIPTION OF THE PROBLEM:

1. Chronology: (When and how did the problem begin?)

2. Under what conditions does vocal cord dysfunction (VCD) occur?

    Exercise: yes / no

    What sports are played?

    VCD is experienced in which sports?

    Circumstances during which VCD occurs: practice   competition

    Non-exercise: yes / no   Under what conditions?

3. Identify symptoms:

    Harder to breathe: in / out / both   Dizziness: yes / no

    Throat tightness: yes / no   Cough: yes / no

    Stridor: yes / no   Numbness/tingling: yes / no

    Rapid breathing: yes / no

4. Rate the usual severity of your attack (circle one):

    Mild—aware of symptoms but continue current activity level

    Moderate—symptoms interfere with activity requiring me to stop and rest

    Severe—symptoms require stopping activity, no sense of control of breathing

    Acute—sought emergency assistance, sense of panic

5. Do you experience breathing problems every time you exercise?   Yes   No

6. Rate the frequency of your attacks (circle one):

    Seldom—rarely happens

    Occasional—happens occasionally when I'm exposed to VCD trigger

    Frequent—happens almost every time I'm exposed to VCD trigger

    Very frequent—happens each time I'm exposed to VCD trigger

7. Can you predict an ensuing attack? What are the first symptoms?

8. Do the symptoms begin suddenly or gradually?

Copyright © 2007 by Mosby, Inc., an affiliate of Elsevier Inc. All rights reserved.

VOCAL CORD DYSFUNCTION, *cont'd*

9. Have you required emergency intervention? If yes, describe.

10. When exercising do you experience repeat episodes within the same work-out session or game?

11. Do asthma medications help reduce or eliminate attacks?

12. Are you currently using asthma medications?

13. What do you do to stop an attack? How long does it take for symptoms to subside?

14. What is your reaction during and following an attack?

II. MEDICAL HISTORY

1. Indicate the specialists that have been consulted for this problem:

   Asthma/Allergist   Pulmonologist   Cardiologist

   ENT   Gastroenterologist   Internist

   Pediatrician   Speech-language pathologist

   Psychologist/Counselor   Other: _____

2. Indicate concurrent medical conditions:

   Asthma ___   Allergies ___

   Reflux (discuss symptoms) ___   Chronic postnasal drip ___

   ADD/ADHD ___   Neurological condition ___

   Habit cough ___   Chronic hoarseness ___

   Psychological problem: Anxiety ___ Depression ___ OCD ___

   Sleep disorder ___

   Other:_____

3. What medications are currently being taken?

4. Describe your overall health. (Typical school/work year, number of absences?)

III. PSYCHOLOGICAL/EDUCATIONAL HISTORY

1. Which of the following words describes you (circle):

   self-motivated   perfectionist   procrastinator

   goal-oriented   good student   positive self-concept

   worrier   anxious   competitive

   Other descriptors: _____

Copyright © 2007 by Mosby, Inc., an affiliate of Elsevier Inc. All rights reserved.

VOCAL CORD DYSFUNCTION, *cont'd*

2. What kinds of things cause you to worry?

3. During the time that this problem began or since its onset, have there been any emotionally troubling events or excessive stress in your life? (divorce; death; family conflict; anxiety about school or sports; increase in competition level)

4. Do you think that stress/nervousness/competition cause or exacerbate your problem? If yes, give an example.

5. Have you had or are you currently involved in psychological evaluation and/or counseling? If so, for what reason?

IV. SPORTS HISTORY (If VCD accompanies sports)

1. Sports played throughout the year

2. Level of competition

3. Practice regimen for current sport(s) where VCD is experienced

4. Long-range athletic goals:

V. EVALUATION

Voice and Larynx:

Quality: WNL   HOARSE   EFFORTFUL   SPASMING
Loudness: WNL
Pitch: WNL
Visual presence of laryngeal tension: _____
Palpable presence of laryngeal tension: _____
Laryngeal/vocal fold structure: _____
Laryngeal/vocal fold function when not symptomatic: _____
Laryngeal/vocal fold function when symptomatic: _____
Method of examination: _____

Respiration:

Maximum phonation duration: sustained /a/: _____ sec _____ sec
Sustained /s/: _____ sec _____ sec
Spirometry measurements: _____
Oxygen saturation: _____
Phonatory airflow: _____ Phonatory air pressure: _____
Observations:

Copyright © 2007 by Mosby, Inc., an affiliate of Elsevier Inc. All rights reserved.

VOCAL CORD DYSFUNCTION, *cont'd*

VI. SAMPLE THERAPY HIERARCHY

1. Discuss normal and paradoxical vocal cord motion during breathing (use model of larynx).

2. View videotape of vocal cord dysfunction.

3. Discuss possible causes.

   Psychogenic   GERD/LPR   Postnasal drip   "Aerobic overload"

4. Teach breathing method. (Goal of method is to control but ultimately prevent an attack.)
   - Teach lengthened exhalation with /s/ or pursed lips
   - Gentle, abdominal inhalation transnasally (shorter than exhale)
   - Teach idea of inhale:exhale ratio and rhythm
   - Release of tension in upper torso, head and neck
   - Positive thinking/imagery/self-talk

5. Transition VCD breathing into exercise (If appropriate).

   Walking   Jogging   Running   Sprinting   Intervals

Rhythmic breathing matching footsteps:	**yes**	**no**
Abdominal breathing vs. upper chest:	**yes**	**no**
Upper torso reduced tension:	**yes**	**no**
Ratio established and altered as needed:	**yes**	**no**

   Comfort level with technique: _____

   Amount of time spent exercising: _____   Distance: _____

   VCD symptoms observed: _____

   Self-report of maximum throat tightness (0 = none vs. 5 = extreme): _____

6. Simulate VCD breathing into other sports (i.e., swimming).

7. Additional techniques taught:

   _____ Inspiratory muscle trainer

   _____ Laryngeal massage

   _____ Other: _____

VII. RECOMMENDATIONS

_____ Chart VCD breathing practice and success with techniques

_____ Practice VCD breathing techniques at rest

_____ Practice VCD breathing techniques while exercising

_____ Recommend additional session(s)

_____ Recommend ENT consultation

_____ Recommend pulmonary consultation

_____ SLP follow-up with referring M.D.

   ___ Request records

   ___ Discuss case

   ___ Suggest counseling

   ___ Suggest additional consults or therapy _____

_____ Discuss case with coach, trainer, guidance counselor

Copyright © 2007 by Mosby, Inc., an affiliate of Elsevier Inc. All rights reserved.

SAMPLE PULMONOLOGY REPORT FOR HABIT COUGH

HISTORY OF PRESENT ILLNESS

Today I saw Michael, a 12-year-old male, for a consultation, having been referred by his pediatrician. Michael has a history of environmental allergies with multiple positive skin tests and has been on immunotherapy for the past 5 years. Four months ago, he developed an upper respiratory infection (URI) and has had a cough since. He has no other associated symptoms with his cough. His cough is a dry, spasmodic cough that varies in frequency and severity from day to day. When his cough starts, many times it will go on for a long time unabated. It does not seem to wake him up at night. In the first hour after he wakes in the morning, he does not seem to cough; then his cough will begin. He has no history of asthma or pneumonia. His growth has been normal. He has no chronic gastrointestinal (GI) symptoms. He has taken Augmentin, Zithromax, Advair, Prednisone, Tessalon, Atrovent, Zyrtec, Claritin, and Delsym without any significant change in his cough.

Birth history, family history, and environmental history are unremarkable. He is on Concerta, Ritalin, and Zoloft for ADHD. He has been on these medications for the past 2 years and is being monitored by a psychiatrist. Mother states that Michael has difficulty with peers and is sometimes bullied.

PHYSICAL EXAMINATION

Respiratory rate 20 and unlabored; weight 135 pounds; height 60 inches. Examination of head, ears, nose, and throat is normal. Lungs are normal. Heart shows a normal rhythm without murmurs. Abdomen is soft; bowel sounds are normal and active, with no masses or tenderness. Skin examination is normal. Extremities are without clubbing, cyanosis, or edema.

Labs Today

Oxygen saturation on room air was 98%. Spirometry measurements: FVC 118% of predicted, FEV_1 121% of predicted, FEF 25-75, 128% of predicted. These results are all supranormal. Sinus CT scan and chest x-ray were normal.

IMPRESSION/PLAN

Michael has a chronic cough and coughed several times during this examination. The character of his cough is typical of a psychogenic or habit cough, and I feel that this is his diagnosis. The only other possibility would be a tic, but I think this is unlikely. He has not responded to any medications, which is quite typical of habit cough. I discussed my findings with his mother and recommended that he see a speech-language pathologist who is highly skilled in dealing with youngsters with habit cough. I also asked mother to follow up with Michael's psychiatrist as soon as possible for any other suggestions that may be helpful. For now I do not feel that any medications are necessary.

Courtesy of Dr. Samuel Rosenberg, M.D., Pediatric Pulmonologist, Pediatric Pulmonary and Asthma Center, Rockville, Md.

Copyright © 2007 by Mosby, Inc., an affiliate of Elsevier Inc. All rights reserved.

HABIT COUGH

PATIENT INTERVIEW

Patient: _____

Address: _____

_____

Phone: _____

Parents (if minor): _____

Date of Eval: _____

Date of Birth: _____

Occupation: _____

E-mail Address: _____

Referring M.D.: _____

I. DESCRIPTION OF THE PROBLEM:

1. Chronology: **When** and **how** did the problem begin?

2. Describe the cough.

   Single cough _____   Repetitive cough _____

   Normal sound _____   Bizarre sound (honk) _____

   Elicits a gag reflex or vomiting _____

   Follows a "tickle" or "itch" feeling _____

3. How long has it persisted?

4. Have there been previous periods of habit cough?

5. What interventions have been tried?

6. What interventions (if any) have been successful?

7. Is cough absent during sleep?

8. Has school (work) been missed? *If yes,* how much time?

9. Is there a daily or activity pattern related to the cough frequency?

10. Are there activities or social situations being avoided because of cough?

11. What is your (the client's) reaction to the problem?

12. What is the reaction of family members, peers, teachers?

Copyright © 2007 by Mosby, Inc., an affiliate of Elsevier Inc. All rights reserved.

HABIT COUGH, *cont'd*

II. MEDICAL HISTORY

1. Did an illness precede the cough? (*If yes,* describe.)

2. Have you been hospitalized for the cough?

3. Discuss chronic and recent illnesses and hospitalizations.

4. What medications are currently being taken?

5. Indicate the specialists that have been consulted for this problem.

   Allergist   Pulmonologist   Neurologist

   ENT   Gastroenterologist

   Pediatrician   Speech-language pathologist

   Psychologist/Counselor   Other: _____

6. Indicate concurrent medical conditions.

   Asthma   Allergies

   Reflux   Chronic postnasal drip

   ADD/ADHD   Neurological condition

   Learning disability   Obsession/Compulsion

   Tourette's syndrome   Anxiety

   Sleep disorder   Depression

   Other:_____

7. Do family members have any of the above conditions?

8. Has your larynx been examined? (*If yes,* discuss method and findings.)

III. SOCIAL EMOTIONAL HISTORY

1. Did a stressful event or stressful time period precede or accompany the cough? (*If yes,* discuss.)

2. Is stress, anxiety, or conflict occurring in your life currently? (*If yes,* discuss.)

3. Describe your (the client's) personality.

4. Describe family, peer, teacher, and work relationships.

5. Describe your school (work) performance.

Copyright © 2007 by Mosby, Inc., an affiliate of Elsevier Inc. All rights reserved.

HABIT COUGH, *cont'd*

IV. EVALUATION

Presence of cough:

Frequency (number of coughs in 10 minutes):

Severity:

Reaction:

Observations: co-occurring behaviors, client affect, family interaction

Presence of excessive laryngeal tension:

Voice: Quality _____ Pitch _____ Loudness _____

Speech:

Language:

V. TREATMENT

___ Gentle abdominal inhalation

___ Lengthened exhalation with /s/

___ Blowing with pursed lips

___ Sipping and swallowing

___ Substituting a different behavior for the cough

Other: _____

Success with techniques:

Length of time cough was controlled while using cough reduction techniques:

Client/Family reaction:

VI. RECOMMENDATIONS

_____ Chart cough frequency and success with techniques

_____ Practice cough management techniques

_____ Follow up via e-mail or phone

_____ Recommend additional session(s)

_____ SLP follow-up with referring M.D.

   ___ Request records

   ___ Discuss case

   ___ Suggest counseling

   ___ Suggest additional consults or therapy _____

Additional Comments:

Copyright © 2007 by Mosby, Inc., an affiliate of Elsevier Inc. All rights reserved.

SIGNS AND SYMPTOMS OF DEPRESSION

1. Depressed (sad, empty) mood most of the day as indicated by self-report or observation; in children and adolescents can be irritable mood
2. Markedly diminished interest or pleasure in all or most all activities, most of the day as indicated by self-report or observation
3. Significant weight loss or gain or significant decrease or increase in appetite
4. Insomnia or hypersomnia
5. Headaches; vague aches and pains; digestive problems; dizziness
6. Neglect of personal grooming
7. Vocal symptoms of monotonicity (flat sounding voice), frequent sighing
8. Frequent unexplained crying
9. Psychomotor agitation (restlessness) or retardation (slowed down), as self reported and observed by others
10. Fatigue or loss of energy
11. Feelings of worthlessness
12. Feelings of isolation/social withdrawal
13. Feelings of inappropriate guilt (not just guilt about being sick)
14. Diminished ability to think, concentrate, or remember
15. Indecisiveness
16. Recurrent thoughts of death, recurrent suicidal ideation with or without a plan, or a suicide attempt

Data from Cymbalta: *Symptoms and causes of depression*, 2005. Retrieved April 20, 2005, from http://www.cymbalta.com/depression/understand/causes.jsp?reqNavId=1.3; National Institute of Mental Health: *Depression*, 2006. Retrieved February 25, 2006, from http://www.nimh.nih.gov/healthinformation/depressionmenu.cfm

Copyright © 2007 by Mosby, Inc., an affiliate of Elsevier Inc. All rights reserved.

TYPES AND SYMPTOMS OF ANXIETY DISORDERS

DIFFERENT TYPES OF ANXIETY DISORDERS

1. **Panic disorder**—repeated episodes of intense fear that occur with little warning, causing physical symptoms such as chest pain, heart palpitations, hyperventilation, dizziness, and feelings of unreality
2. **Obsessive-compulsive disorder**—repeated, unwanted thoughts or behaviors for which the person feels no control
3. **Social phobia**—a disabling fear of being criticized, humiliated, or embarrassed in social situations that causes avoidance of these situations
4. **Specific phobia**—extreme, irrational fear of something that poses little actual danger, but leads to avoidance of objects or situations
5. **Posttraumatic stress syndrome**—persistent frightening thoughts and adverse physical symptoms following exposure to a terrifying event or situation in which physical harm occurred or was threatened
6. **Generalized anxiety disorder**—constant, exaggerated, unrealistic worry about everyday life events and activities, lasting at least 6 months, accompanied by physical symptoms such as muscle tension

SYMPTOMS OF GENERALIZED ANXIETY DISORDER

1. Excessive anxiety and worry (apprehensive expectation) occurring more days than not, about events or activities (such as work or school performance or health related events)
2. Difficulty controlling the worry
3. Restlessness or feeling keyed up or on edge; heart palpitations
4. Fatigue or loss of energy
5. Diminished ability to think, concentrate, or remember
6. Irritability
7. Muscle tension and pain; headaches; tense facial expression, and body posture
8. Sleep disturbance (difficulty falling or staying asleep, or restless sleep)
9. Gastrointestinal problems

Data from National Institute of Mental Health: *Anxiety disorders*, 2006. Retrieved February 25, 2006, from http://www.nimh.nih.gov/healthinformation/anxietymenu.cfm; Psych Central: *Facts about anxiety disorders*, 1999. Retrieved April 20, 2005, from http://www.psychcentral.com/disorders/anxietyfacts.htm

Copyright © 2007 by Mosby, Inc., an affiliate of Elsevier Inc. All rights reserved.

TREATMENT

Exciting things are happening in the profession of speech-language pathology as it relates to therapy. "Evidence-based practice" has made this profession more accountable than ever in the service delivery models and therapy techniques.[1,62] The area of voice disorders is no exception.[55] A book this size cannot present a comprehensive overview of therapy, but there are many fine texts that do that.

The therapy portion of this book is intended to give the SLP some needed tools to effectively plan and execute therapy. The "ASHA Preferred Practice Patterns"[5] for voice intervention appear first to give the SLP an understanding of the expectations for providing therapy for voice, resonance, and laryngeal disorders. The next information addresses areas of treatment that the author has observed as being especially challenging to graduate students and newly practicing clinicians. This includes developing goals, planning therapy, constructing treatment hierarchies, documenting progress, and reporting results. Armed with this practical information, in concert with a comprehensive text, I've seen many student clinicians have an "ah hah!" experience, as they begin to grasp the gestalt of voice therapy.

The chart devoted to goal development (see pages 145-146), created by Mary M. Klimek, M.M., M.S., CCC/SLP Voice and Speech Laboratory, Massachusetts Eye and Ear Infirmary, offers incredible utility to the SLP by providing measurable long-term, short-term, and treatment session goal ideas. The reader is able to cut and paste from pull-down menus (figuratively speaking) to construct goals for most any laryngeal and voice disorder. Taking data for voice goals can be challenging, thus the student is encouraged to use the varying methods that are provided in this section (performance assessments as well as individual, norm, and criterion referenced measures) to assess client performance throughout the treatment process. The form that is provided for documenting the treatment session follows a SOAP (subjective, objective, assessment, and plan) format but is very inclusive for perceptual and acoustic documentation (see page 151). It also functions well for reporting diagnostic results.

Because the author has had quite extensive experience in vocal cord dysfunction and habit cough treatment, the therapy techniques and materials found to be effective with these disorders are included. In addition, diagrams illustrating the components needed for a well-balanced voice and the art of laryngeal massage have been included because they have proven to be extremely valuable tools for client education, encouraging insightful feedback, particularly in the area of muscle tension dysphonia (MTD).

The other materials included in this section are educational resources for the client and/or clinician on topics such as voice care, reflux, and counseling tips.

Copyright © 2007 by Mosby, Inc., an affiliate of Elsevier Inc. All rights reserved.

ASHA 2004 PREFERRED PRACTICE PATTERNS FOR THE PROFESSION OF SPEECH-LANGUAGE PATHOLOGY

#35. VOICE INTERVENTION

Intervention services are provided for individuals with voice disorders, alaryngeal speech, and/or laryngeal disorder affecting respiration, including possible organic, neurologic, behavioral, and psychosocial etiologies.

Intervention is conducted consistent with the *Fundamental Components and Guiding Principles*.

Individuals Who Provide the Services

Voice interventions are conducted by appropriately credentialed and trained speech-language pathologists, possibly supported by speech-language pathology assistants under appropriate supervision.

Expected Outcomes

Consistent with the World Health Organization (WHO) framework, intervention is designed to—

- Capitalize on strengths and address weaknesses related to underlying structures and functions that affect voice production;
- Facilitate the individual's activities and participation by assisting the person to acquire new communication skills and strategies;
- Modify contextual factors to reduce barriers and enhance facilitators of successful communication and participation, and to provide appropriate accommodations and other supports, as well as training in how to use them.

Intervention is conducted to achieve improved voice production, coordination of respiration and laryngeal valving, and/or acquisition of alaryngeal speech sufficient to allow for functional oral communication.

Intervention is expected to result in improved abilities, functioning, participation, and contextual facilitators. Intervention also may result in recommendations for reassessment or follow-up, or in a referral for other services.

Clinical Indications

Voice intervention is prompted by the results of a voice assessment. Individuals of all ages receive treatment and/or consultation services when their ability to communicate effectively is impaired because of a voice disorder and when there is a reasonable expectation of benefit to the individual in body structure/function and/or activity/participation. Interventions that enhance activity and participation through modification of contextual factors may be warranted even if the prognosis for improved body structure/function is limited.

Clinical Process

Intervention involves providing timely information and guidance to patients/clients, families, and significant persons about the nature of voice disorders, alaryngeal speech, and/or laryngeal disorders affecting respiration; and the goals, procedures, respective responsibilities, and the likely outcome of treatment.

Depending on assessment results, intervention addresses the following:

- The individual's preferences, goals, and special needs to enhance participation and improve functioning in life activities that the individual and family and relevant others deem important.
- Appropriate voice care and conservation guidelines, including strategies that promote healthy laryngeal tissues and voice production and reduce laryngeal trauma or strain.

Copyright © 2007 by Mosby, Inc., an affiliate of Elsevier Inc. All rights reserved.

- Proper use of respiratory, phonatory, and resonatory processes to achieve improved voice production, coordination of respiration and laryngeal valving, with appropriate treatment to enhance these behaviors.
- Patient/client-directed selection of preferred alaryngeal speech communication means, including development of one or more of the following alaryngeal alternatives: esophageal speech, artificial larynx speech, or tracheoesophageal prosthesis speech.
- Materials and approaches appropriate to the individual's chronological and developmental age, medical status, physical and sensory abilities, education, vocation, cognitive status, and cultural, socioeconomic, and linguistic backgrounds.
- Assistance with a voice disorder, alaryngeal speech, and/or laryngeal disorder that affects respiration to maintain treatment targets in oral communication in life activities.
- Follow-up, including interdisciplinary referrals, for other speech and health problems that may accompany the voice disorder, alaryngeal speech, and/or laryngeal disorder affecting respiration, such as medical concerns, dysarthria, swallowing difficulty, emotional disturbance, and other problems.

Intervention is long enough to accomplish stated objectives/predicted outcomes. The intervention period does not continue when there is no longer any expectation for further benefit.

Setting, Equipment Specifications, Safety and Health Precautions

SETTING: Intervention may be conducted in a variety of settings, including clinical, educational, and other natural environments that are selected on the basis of intervention goals and in considerations of the social, academic, and/or vocational activities that are relevant to or desired by the individual. In any setting, intervention addresses the personal and environmental factors that are barriers to or facilitators of the patient's/client's voice production. There is a plan to generalize and maintain intervention gains and to increase participation in relevant settings and activities.

EQUIPMENT SPECIFICATIONS: When available, instrumental measures may be used in treatment to monitor progress and to provide appropriate patient/client feedback of voice production and/or laryngeal function. Instrumental techniques ensure the validity of signal processing, analysis routines, and elimination of task or signal artifacts. All equipment is used and maintained in accordance with the manufacturer's specifications.

SAFETY AND HEALTH PRECAUTIONS: All procedures ensure the safety of the patient/client and clinician and adhere to universal health precautions (e.g., prevention of bodily injury and transmission of infectious disease).

Laryngeal imaging techniques and selection/placement of tracheoesophageal prostheses are conducted in settings that have access to emergency medical treatment, if needed.

Decontamination, cleaning, disinfection, and sterilization of multiple-use equipment before reuse are carried out according to facility-specific infection control policies and procedures and according to the manufacturer's instructions.

Documentation

Documentation includes the following:
- Written record of the dates, length, and type of interventions that were provided.
- Progress toward stated goals, updated prognosis, and specific recommendations.
- Evaluation of intervention outcomes and effectiveness within the WHO framework of body structures/functions, activities/participation, and contextual factors.

The privacy and security of documentation are maintained in compliance with the regulations of the Health Insurance Portability and Accountability Act (HIPAA), Family Educational Rights and Privacy Act (FERPA), and other state and federal laws.

Copyright © 2007 by Mosby, Inc., an affiliate of Elsevier Inc. All rights reserved.

ASHA Policy Documents and Selected References

American Speech-Language-Hearing Association. (1993). Position statement and guidelines for oral and oropharyngeal prostheses. *ASHA, 35*(Suppl. 10), 14–16.

American Speech-Language-Hearing Association. (1993). Position statement and guidelines on the use of voice prostheses in tracheotomized persons with or without ventilatory dependence. *ASHA, 35*(Suppl. 10), 17–20.

American Speech-Language-Hearing Association. (2004). Evaluation and treatment for tracheoesophageal puncture and prosthesis: Technical report. *ASHA Supplement 24*, 166–177.

American Speech-Language-Hearing Association. (2004). Knowledge and skills for speech-language pathologists with respect to evaluation and treatment for tracheoesophageal puncture and prosthesis. *ASHA Supplement 24*, 166–177.

American Speech-Language-Hearing Association. (2004). Knowledge and skills for speech-language pathologists with respect to vocal tract visualization and imaging. *ASHA Supplement 24*, 184–192.

American Speech-Language-Hearing Association. (2004). Roles and responsibilities of speech-language pathologists with respect to evaluation and treatment for tracheoesophageal puncture and prosthesis. *ASHA Supplement 24*, 63.

American Speech-Language-Hearing Association. (2004). Vocal tract visualization and imaging: Position statement. *ASHA Supplement 24*, 64.

American Speech-Language-Hearing Association. (2004). Vocal tract visualization and imaging: Technical report. *ASHA Supplement 24*, 135–139.

World Health Organization. (2001). *International classification of functioning, disability and health*. Geneva, Switzerland: Author.

From American Speech-Language- Hearing Association: *Preferred practice patterns for the profession of speech-language pathology*, 2004. Retrieved February 28, 2005, from http://www.asha.org/members/deskref-journal/deskref/default

Copyright © 2007 by Mosby, Inc., an affiliate of Elsevier Inc. All rights reserved.

GUIDELINES FOR VOICE THERAPY

SUCCESSFUL VOICE THERAPY DEPENDS UPON:

1. An accurate medical diagnosis
2. An accurate voice diagnosis
3. An appropriate treatment plan
4. Clinician and client agreement regarding the diagnosis, treatment plan, and expected outcome
5. A commitment by the client or the family (when a child), to address the problem
6. Self-discipline by the client (or support system) to make necessary behavioral changes

TREATMENT PLANNING: QUESTIONS CLINICIANS NEED TO ASK THEMSELVES

1. What am I teaching the client? (Specific goals and treatment techniques that will change the voice)
   a. Is the technique applicable and appropriate for this client with this problem?
   b. Can I explain the technique and its rationale?
   c. Can I model the technique?
   d. Can I make the client feel comfortable when he or she is trying the "strange" techniques?
2. How will I know if therapy is successful?
   a. What perceptual change can I expect?
   b. Will the change be a gradual one or immediate?
   c. What acoustic (measurable) changes can I expect?
   d. What stroboscopic/physiological changes can I expect?
   e. What aerodynamic findings can I expect?
   f. What information might the client give that indicates success?
3. What will the progression of therapy (or a given technique) be?
   a. A hierarchy needs to be developed to move the client from point A to point Z.
   b. Advance preparation is needed whether the client is ready to make great leaps, make small steps, or regress.
   c. The clinician must have a knowledge base that includes:
      i. Many facilitative techniques (especially those with efficacy data)
      ii. A plan for progression from one technique to another
      iii. Recognition for when to discontinue a technique
4. What materials are needed for each technique? (How can materials and techniques be adapted to children?)
   a. Since drill is often mandatory, how can it be made interesting and functional?
   b. Since homework is needed, what should an assignment consist of?
5. How will I take data?
   a. Refer to this book for suggestions.
   b. If possible, gather both acoustic and perceptual data to obtain clearer results.
6. How can I effectively reinforce the client's behavior?
   a. Are the comments that I make meaningful, helpful, and accurate?
   b. Do I need tangible reinforcement?
   c. Am I using recording playback or visual feedback in a meaningful way?
7. How will I know when to terminate therapy?
   a. When the treatment goals have been met
   b. When dictated by insurance
   c. When the client is satisfied with the therapy outcome
   d. When progress has reached a plateau or there is a lack of compliance
   e. When further medical, surgical, or psychosocial treatment is indicated

Copyright © 2007 by Mosby, Inc., an affiliate of Elsevier Inc. All rights reserved.

A GUIDE FOR FORMULATING GOALS FOR VOICE AND LARYNGEAL TREATMENT

The patient/client will... *(Complete with appropriate selections.)*

(A) PERFORMANCE	(B) CRITERION ATTRIBUTES
Education Lifestyle Vocal Hygiene Implement reflux management recommendations Implement vocal hygiene recommendations Keep a voice use journal to identify ± vocal behaviors Drink ___ or more ounces of water Demonstrate knowledge of the basics of voice production Substitute swallow/silent cough for voiced throat clear/cough **Relaxation** Perform relaxation exercises Perform laryngeal massage Perform stretching exercises **Breathing** Pant Candle-blow (__ sustained/ ___ pulsed) Hiss (__ sustained/ ___ pulsed) Use abdominal/low thoracic breathing patterns Coordinate breath with phrasing Coordinate breath with exercise **Voice and Resonance** Speak Speak 3 syllables per breath Speak 3-5 syllables per breath Speak 5-8 syllables per breath Speak 8-12 syllables per breath Produce resonant, relaxed voice Perform relaxation, breathing, and voice exercises to recondition voice **TX Programs** Complete LSVT home program Demonstrate weekly improvement in duration/range/intensity of LSVT tasks Demonstrate carryover of "think loud/think shout" strategy Complete vocal function exercises Demonstrate weekly improvement in range/duration of VFE's Complete resonant voice therapy home exercises **Alaryngeal Speech** Produce esophageal voice-inhalation; prephonation; consonant injection Reduce auditory and visual distracters accompanying voice Produce voice via tracheoesophageal puncture Coordinate sound generation of artificial larynx and articulation Practice speech production drills with electrolarynx	**General** Accurately Correctly Adequately Optimally With ease Comfortably Rhythmically Steadily Slowly **Re: Voicing** With increased stability Without voice breaks With clear tone With near-clear tone With improved tone With reduced effort With easy voice onsets With abrupt voice onsets With appropriate loudness With appropriate pitch With appropriate breath support With resonant tone Without vocal fry Using facilitative technique **Re: Overall Production** With appropriate balance of oral/nasal resonance With increased pitch/loudness inflections With appropriate rate Without losing breath connection Without fatigue Without visible strain/tension With intelligibility With feminine attributes With masculine attributes With even/steady breath flow rate With appropriate range of lung volume **Alaryngeal Speech** With intelligibility to family members With intelligibility to unfamiliar listeners

Copyright © 2007 by Mosby, Inc., an affiliate of Elsevier Inc. All rights reserved.

A GUIDE FOR FORMULATING GOALS FOR VOICE AND LARYNGEAL TREATMENT, *cont'd*

(C) CONSISTENCY	(D) COMPLEXITY	(E) CONDITIONS/CUING
For 5 repetitions	In kazoo buzzes	In quiet environments
For 10 repetitions	In voiced lip/tongue trills	In controlled environments
For ___ repetitions	In "raspberries"	In public spaces
	During speaking range pitch glides	On the telephone
QD (daily)	During maximum range pitch glides	At home (by self/other's report)
BID (2 times/day)	In vowel prolongations	At work/school
TID (3 times/day)	In sustained phonation of comfortable duration	With spouse
	In sustained phonation of maximum duration	With caregivers
10% of the time	While completing all vocal tasks	
20% of the time		While walking briskly
30% of the time	In single-syllable word lists	While exercising
40% of the time	In 1-3–syllable word lists	With masking
50% of the time	In short phrases (3-5 syllables)	With delayed auditory feedback
60% of the time	In 5-10–syllable phrases and sentences	With minimal background noise
70% of the time	In 10-15–syllable phrases and sentences	With moderate background noise
80% of the time	In 3-8–syllable W and Y initial practice phrases	With extreme background noise
90% of the time	In 3-8–syllable M/N initial practice phrases	
100% of the time	In 3-8–syllable H initial practice phrases	Independently
	In 3-8–syllable ___ loaded practice phrases	With intermittent cues/models
5 of 7 days of the week	In vowel-initial words and short phrases	With instructional cues only
6 of 7 days of the week		With min cues
For 4 weeks running		With min-mod cues
Throughout treatment period	While reciting phrases and sentences	With mod cues
	While reciting aloud	With mod-max cues
For 5 minutes		With max cues
For 10 minutes	In oral reading tasks (paragraphs and articles)	
For 15 minutes	While answering open-ended question	On topic of personal interest
For 20 minutes	In monologues	With emotionally charged topic
For 25 minutes	In structured conversations	
For 30 minutes	When speaking spontaneously	
For 45 minutes	In conversational speech	
For 50 minutes		
For 55 minutes		
For 60 minutes		

Created by Mary M. Klimek, M.M., M.S., CCC/SLP and Clinical Staff at Voice and Speech Laboratory, Massachusetts Eye and Ear Infirmary.

Copyright © 2007 by Mosby, Inc., an affiliate of Elsevier Inc. All rights reserved.

A SAMPLE HIERARCHY FOR MASK FOCUS

A TREATMENT TECHNIQUE FOR VOCAL HYPERFUNCTION

I. Establishment of sound and feel of voice in the "mask" of the face

Prolonged nasal sounds

Humming

Nasalized "uh hum"

II. Prolonged nasal sounds in single syllables

me	*my*
may	*mow*
ma	*more*
knee	*no*

III. Prolonged nasal sounds in single syllable words

meet	*mine*
make	*mowed*
mop	*march*
move	*mad*
nose	*neat*

IV. Prolonged nasal sounds in multisyllabic words

meter	*myself*
maybe	*Monday*
model	*marble*
movie	*matches*
never	*neighbor*

V. Nasal sounds in phrases (Prolong as needed to maintain feel of mask focus.)

Monday morning

Mine is not

Maybe later

Me too

My house

VI. Nasal sounds in phrases with normal articulation and prosody (Therapist asks the following questions and client answers with the phrases from V.)

When is your appointment?	*Monday morning*
My dinner is good, what about yours?	*Mine is not*
Are you going?	*Maybe later*
I'm exhausted, how about you?	*Me too*
Where is the party?	*My house*

Copyright © 2007 by Mosby, Inc., an affiliate of Elsevier Inc. All rights reserved.

VII. Nasal sounds in sentences of increasing length (Prolong nasal sound as needed to maintain feel of mask focus.)

Meet me at school.

Monopoly is fun.

My mailman comes by noon.

My mother makes great meals.

Mr. McNew is never on time.

Millions of ants marched onto the blanket.

More and more technology is made.

VIII. Nasal sounds in meaningful speech (Prolong nasal sound, hum, or quietly say "uh hum" to achieve mask focus.)

My name _____

My address is _____

My phone number is _____

My occupation is _____

My hobbies are _____

My birthday is _____

My favorite food is _____

IX. Maintenance of target voice in longer speech with varying phonemes, using /m/ or "uh hum" as reminders of mask focus

Days of the week

Months of the year

Counting

Reciting the alphabet

Pledge of Allegiance

Memorized poems, prayers, song lyrics

X. Reading material of increasing length

Newspapers	*Trivia books*
Magazines	*Professional materials of the client's*
Children's books	*Bible*

Copyright © 2007 by Mosby, Inc., an affiliate of Elsevier Inc. All rights reserved.

XI. Monologues with topics requiring thought or emotion (Hum, or quietly say "uh hum" to achieve or regain mask focus.)

> *Tell me how to get from your home to the nearest grocery store (park, etc.).*
>
> *Describe your kitchen (desk, pet, etc.).*
>
> *Discuss your favorite hobby (TV show, restaurant, etc.).*
>
> *Describe a person whom you admire.*
>
> *Tell why you sought voice therapy and your impression of it.*

XII. Conversational exchange with the clinician or others (Think or say "uh hum" to achieve or regain mask focus as needed.)

Data from Cooper M: *Stop committing voice suicide*, Los Angeles, 1996, Voice & Speech Company of America; Lessac A: *The use and training of the human voice*, New York, 1973, Drama Book Specialists.

Copyright © 2007 by Mosby, Inc., an affiliate of Elsevier Inc. All rights reserved.

METHODS FOR EVALUATING CLIENTS' PERFORMANCE

I. Performance assessment
   A. ± Good voice/poor voice rating
   B. Number rating scale (*example:* 3-point interval scale)
      1. Clear or best voice
      2. Improved voice/negative feature reduced
      3. Poor voice
   C. Length of time target voice is maintained
   D. Reduction in frequency of a specific behavior during or outside of therapy (*example:* phonation breaks, coughs, etc.) through keeping a tally
   E. Client effort rating scale (*example:* 3-point interval scale)
      1. No/low laryngeal effort felt when producing voice
      2. Moderate laryngeal effort felt
      3. Excessive laryngeal effort felt
   F. Anecdotal reports from the client and from listeners
II. Individualized referenced measures
   A. Repeat ratings using instruments such as vocal abuse rating scale; reflux symptom index; voice handicap index
   B. Repeated readings or recitation of the same material recorded each therapy session (*example:* "Rainbow Passage," CAPE-V, nursery rhyme) perceptually rated by the clinician using CAPE-V score system
   C. Visual real-time feedback provided by computerized instrumentation
   D. Acoustic analysis, documenting change in target areas (*example:* reduction in frequency perturbation; increase in phonation range; increased MPD)
   E. Improved appearance of the vocal folds through laryngeal examination
III. Norm-referenced measures
   Comparison of client's performance to norm-referenced measures through objective assessment such as SFF, phonation range, perturbation, MPD, intensity, airflow measures
IV. Criterion-referenced measures
   Meeting specified treatment goals

Data from Lanter E: Basics of standardized testing, part III: many ways to evaluate progress, *Adv Speech-Language Pathol* 15(35):4-5, 2005.

CAPE-V, Consensus auditory-perceptual evaluation of voice; *MPD,* maximum phonation duration; *SFF,* speaking fundamental frequency.

Copyright © 2007 by Mosby, Inc., an affiliate of Elsevier Inc. All rights reserved.

DEPARTMENT OF SPEECH-LANGUAGE PATHOLOGY
VOICE THERAPY PROGRESS NOTE

Client's Name: _____   Date of Appointment: _____

Diagnosis: _____   Date last seen: _____

Clinician: _____   Signature: _____

S:

O:

Voice Profile

CAPE-V **Overall Severity** ____ **/100**	
___ rough ___ breathy ___ strained ___ aphonic ___ glottal fry	
___ glottal attacks ___ voice breaks consistent inconsistent	
mild = 1; mild-moderate = 2; moderate = 3; moderate-severe = 4; severe = 5	
Fo Perturbation /a/	
SFF /a/	**SFF—counting**
Optimal Fo /m/	
Fo range	**Number of whole tones**
Loudness	
MPD /a/	
S/Z ratio	

Vocal Abuse

Shouting/yelling/screaming	Singing
Loud talking	Making noises
Talking over noise	Throat clearing
Overall talking	Other:

0 = none; 1 = seldom; 2 = sometimes; 3 = often; 4 = very often; 5 = always.

Vocal Hygiene

water	reflux (RSI score):
medications	stress
caffeine	health
smoke	diet/sleep/exercise

Voice Handicap Index (VHI)

TOTAL SCORE ____ /120	Physical ____ /40	Emotional ____ /40	Functional ____ /40

Copyright © 2007 by Mosby, Inc., an affiliate of Elsevier Inc. All rights reserved.

VOICE THERAPY PROGRESS NOTE, *cont'd*

A:

P:

Copyright © 2007 by Mosby, Inc., an affiliate of Elsevier Inc. All rights reserved.

ESSENTIAL COMPONENTS FOR A WELL-BALANCED VOICE

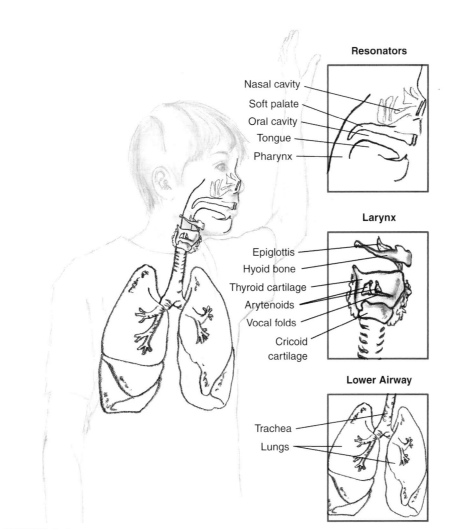

Resonators

Nasal cavity
Soft palate
Oral cavity
Tongue
Pharynx

Larynx

Epiglottis
Hyoid bone
Thyroid cartilage
Arytenoids
Vocal folds
Cricoid
cartilage

Lower Airway

Trachea
Lungs

FIGURE 3-1

Copyright © 2007 by Mosby, Inc., an affiliate of Elsevier Inc. All rights reserved.

NOTES

LARYNGEAL PALPATION AND MASSAGE

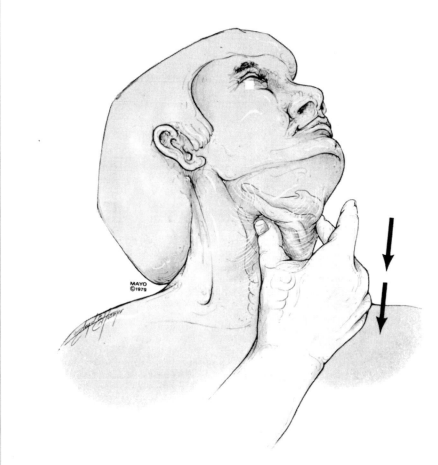

FIGURE 3-2

By permission of Mayo Foundation for Medical Education and Research. All rights reserved.

Copyright © 2007 by Mosby, Inc., an affiliate of Elsevier Inc. All rights reserved.

TREATMENT FOR VOCAL CORD DYSFUNCTION

VCD BREATHING STRATEGY

1. STAY CALM—Focus on your breath out (exhalation)

Use positive self talk and relaxing imagery

2. Begin "VCD breathing"

a. Gentle, short "belly" breath in

b. Longer breath out, using a hissing sound or pursed lips

c. Get into a consistent breathing rhythm in which exhalation is longer than inhalation

3. Reminders:

a. Relax and open your throat (like yawning)

b. Relax your upper body, neck, shoulders, jaw, and tongue

c. Inhale from your belly, not your upper chest

d. Breathe in through your nose if possible (like sniffing)

e. Do not hold your breath

f. If exercising, match your breathing rhythm and inhalation to exhalation ratio to your footsteps (running) or stroke (swimming)

4. Use VCD breathing:

a. Prior to exercising, when warming up or meditating

b. When the first symptom is felt that suggests a VCD episode may occur

c. While exercising (running) or when there is a break in the activity level (field or court sport)

d. During an attack, to reduce the severity and length of the attack

NOTES:

Copyright © 2007 by Mosby, Inc., an affiliate of Elsevier Inc. All rights reserved.

TREATMENT FOR HABIT COUGH: A PLAN FOR THE SLP

COGNITIVE THERAPY

1. Discuss the diagnosis of habit cough with the client and family.
2. Discuss that a habit is a learned behavior, capable of being unlearned.
3. Discuss with the parent (or client) that there is usually a trigger for cough onset.
4. Probe with the client (or parent) possible medical, social, psychological, and academic triggers.

BEHAVIOR MODIFICATION THERAPY[13]

1. Teach behaviors incompatible with coughing:

    a. *Blowing slowly through pursed lips—like blowing a bubble wand*

    b. *Swallowing hard with a "klunk" or slowly with a squeeze*

    c. *Whistling, humming, or talking*

    d. *Gentle or "voiceless" throat clear[75]*

2. Reinforce target (positive) behavior while simultaneously ignoring the cough or reinforcing a reduced frequency of cough through charting.
3. Teach behaviors as substitutes for coughing:

    a. *Inhale gently (vs. deep breath) using diaphragmatic breathing*

    b. *Use a manipulative to squeeze as a response to the cough urge*

4. Introduce desensitization therapy to promote carry-over.

    a. *Determine what behaviors, key words, or topics cause an increase in cough frequency*

    b. *Discuss the observations with the client*

    c. *Purposefully expose the client to the triggers, whereby he or she must refrain from coughing or use another behavior.*

NOTES:

Copyright © 2007 by Mosby, Inc., an affiliate of Elsevier Inc. All rights reserved.

COUGH MANAGEMENT CHART

DATE: _____

Time of Day	Sunday	Monday	Tuesday	Wednesday	Thursday	Friday	Saturday
	C T	C T	C T	C T	C T	C T	C T
	C T	C T	C T	C T	C T	C T	C T
	C T	C T	C T	C T	C T	C T	C T

DIRECTIONS: Pick 3 times during the day when you cough a lot. Write down the time. Monitor your coughing for 10- to 30-minute periods. Use your cough control technique during that period of time. Write down how many times you coughed (C) and how many times you used your technique or trick (T) instead of coughing. The more you practice, the more tallies should appear under the T, and the fewer under the C.

Copyright © 2007 by Mosby, Inc., an affiliate of Elsevier Inc. All rights reserved.

VOICE CARE TIPS

1. Drink water frequently throughout the day.
2. Limit your caffeine and alcohol consumption, because both dry the tissues of the mouth and larynx.
3. Avoid primary or secondary exposure to smoke.
4. Avoid throat clearing and coughing. Try sipping fluids in response to the urge to cough or clear the throat.
5. Avoid yelling, talking at excessive loudness levels, and talking over competing noise because these require maximum effort from the vocal cords.
6. Reduce overall voice use and especially loud voice use during times when you have an upper respiratory infection. Your vocal cords are most susceptible to injury during such times.
7. Be aware of the symptoms of acid reflux, and discuss treatment options with your physician.
8. Attempt to maintain a healthy lifestyle with regard to rest, diet, exercise, and stress management.
9. After speaking for prolonged periods at elevated loudness levels, allow your voice to recover through conservative voice use and increased fluid intake.
10. If you notice a negative change in your voice that lasts longer than 2 weeks, consult your physician.
11. Discuss any medications that you may be taking (prescription or over-the-counter) with your physician to determine whether they are irritating or dehydrating to the vocal cords.
12. If the environment where you work, live, travel, etc. is dry, compensate by drinking more noncaffeinated fluids or using a room humidifier.

NOTES:

Copyright © 2007 by Mosby, Inc., an affiliate of Elsevier Inc. All rights reserved.

LARYNGOPHARYNGEAL REFLUX INFORMATION

SYMPTOMS

1. Chronic coughing and/or throat clearing more bothersome after eating or at night
2. A hoarse voice
3. A feeling of a lump in the throat
4. Excessive nose and throat mucous drainage
5. A sour or bitter taste or burning in the back of the throat
6. A burning sensation below or behind the breast bone (heartburn)
7. Difficulty swallowing or a choking feeling

CAUSE

A weakness in the valve between the stomach and the esophagus causing stomach acid to backflow into the esophagus, larynx, and pharynx (throat).

TREATMENT

1. Consult your pediatrician, family practitioner, or otolaryngologist (ENT) to discuss the use of over-the-counter antacids and prescription medications.
2. Eat small, frequent meals.
3. Reduce your consumption of fatty foods, caffeinated drinks, alcoholic beverages, tomato products, citrus juices, spicy foods, mints, and cigarettes.
4. Sit upright, stand or walk after eating to help keep stomach acid from backing up into the esophagus.
5. Raise the head of your bed 6 inches, or use a wedge-shaped pillow between your mattress and box spring.
6. Don't snack within 3 hours before bedtime.
7. Lose weight if you are overweight.
8. Stay away from garments that are tight fitting around the waist, such as belts or tight jeans.
9. Avoid food or drinks that contain a lot of air such as whipped cream or sodas.

Data from Belafsky P, Postma G, Koufman J: Validity and reliability of the reflux symptom index (RSI), *J Voice* 16(2):274-277, 2002; Rammage L, Morrison M, Nichol H, et al: *Management of the voice and its disorders*, ed 2, Vancouver, Canada, 2001, Singular.

Copyright © 2007 by Mosby, Inc., an affiliate of Elsevier Inc. All rights reserved.

SOURCES OF CAFFEINE*

1. Coffee (7-oz serving)
   115-175 mg drip brew
   .04 mg decaffeinated
2. Tea
   30-70 mg—brewed (7-oz serving)
   16-32 mg—12-oz canned iced tea
3. Soda (12-oz serving)
   55 mg—Mountain Dew
   51 mg—Mello Yello
   41 mg—Sunkist Orange
   41 mg—Dr. Pepper
   37 mg—Pepsi
   364 mg—Diet Pepsi
   34 mg—Coca Cola
   45 mg—Diet Coke
   0 mg—Sprite, 7-Up, Fanta Orange, Hires Root Beer
4. Chocolate
   5 mg—cup of cocoa
   10 mg—1.4 oz milk chocolate bar
   28 mg—1.4 oz dark chocolate bar
5. Nonprescription drugs
   Stimulants (standard dose)
   200 mg—NoDoz
   200 mg—Vivarin
   Pain relievers (standard dose)
   64 mg—Anacin
   130 mg—Excedrin
   65 mg—Midol
   Cold remedies (standard dose)
   32 mg—Dristan
   30 mg—Triaminicin

---

*Average recommended daily intake of caffeine—200 mg

Data from Lopez-Ortiz A: *Frequently asked questions about coffee and caffeine*, 1994.
Retrieved February 27, 2006, from http://www.ameribev.org/industry-issues/healthy-balanced-diet/beverage-ingredients/caffeine/fact-sheets/index.aspx

Copyright © 2007 by Mosby, Inc., an affiliate of Elsevier Inc. All rights reserved.

COUNSELING TIPS FOR THE SLP*

- **Speech-language pathologists need counseling skills.**
  - Communication problems cause psychological issues
    Example: Total laryngectomy
  - Psychological issues cause communication problems
    Example: MTD of psychogenic etiology
  - Communication problems may be a small part of a much bigger problem
    Example: Traumatic brain injury
- **What is the SLP's role regarding psychological intervention?**
  - To listen attentively; to observe the "whole" person; to ask questions
  - To attempt to discern whether counseling is indicated (erring toward intervention)
  - To act immediately if the person talks of taking his own life or the life of another
- **What counseling qualities are needed by the SLP?**
  - To be genuine, honest, accepting and nonjudgmental
  - To be an active, empathic listener—verbally and nonverbally
  - To exercise patience—the SLP is the expert in talking with the communicatively impaired
  - To avoid "Why" type questions; negatively phrased questions (i.e., "You don't lose your temper with your child, do you?"); yes/no questions (instead, pose open-ended ones)
  - To refrain from using personal examples, unless they have very specific relevance
  - To refrain from trying to "fix" the situation (It is much more effective to lead the client and family in forming their own appropriate plans or conclusions.)
  - To recognize the importance of the issue(s), and not trivialize them (Many of our clients and families are going through life-altering events.)

---

*References 23, 39.

SLP, Speech-language pathologist; *MTD,* muscle tension dysphonia.

Copyright © 2007 by Mosby, Inc., an affiliate of Elsevier Inc. All rights reserved.

PART IV

LEARNING OPPORTUNITIES

OVERVIEW

With the advent of the Knowledge and Skill Assessment (KASA), new teaching models clearly pointed toward helping students merge academic knowledge with clinical skills and assessments. To this author, who functions as classroom instructor and clinical supervisor, it signaled the end of traditional classroom lecture format and the beginning of creative teaching and learning models. One such change was the institution of four labs that were completed throughout the semester, as they coincided with the course curriculum, focusing on respiration, voice, resonation, and alaryngeal speech. The challenge was to create simulations of clinician/client dyads that could be completed in approximately 1 hour of class time per lab, with a minimum of instrumentation and equipment being needed. The labs that follow in this section are samples of those four labs—to be completed along with the appropriate course material. The intent of these labs is to teach basic concepts and stretch thinking skills through hands-on learning.

The reader will note that for each lab, the specific ASHA standards from the KASA have been included. This will aid the instructor in ensuring and documenting that these standards are being taught in the classroom setting. Following the ASHA standards, materials and equipment needed for the lab are listed. Depending on the university or facility where the labs are conducted, the equipment and materials can be increased in sophistication as deemed appropriate by the instructor. At the end of each lab, there is a section for additional research and discussion. This section was created primarily as a source that could be used for student remediation, if class or clinic performance has warranted it. (If the reader is unfamiliar with the remediation process, refer to ASHA guidelines for graduate student training.) After student completion of the lab exercise, the instructor should engage the classroom in a rich discussion regarding the topics covered in the lab; in that way, any questions the student may have can be addressed.

Each lab is available on the accompanying CD. By requiring students to submit the labs for graded instructor evaluation, students are motivated to stay focused on the tasks covered in these labs.

Copyright © 2007 by Mosby, Inc., an affiliate of Elsevier Inc. All rights reserved.

Respiration Lab*

ASHA CERTIFICATION STANDARDS ADDRESSED: III-B, III-C, III-D

MATERIALS NEEDED: Watch with second hand, copy of Rainbow Passage (see page 111), tape recorder (optional)

Name: _____ Partner: _____ Date: _____

I. **Nonspeech breathing**

   A. Sitting in a comfortable relaxed position, count the number of breaths you take in 1 minute. Record the number: _____ These are referred to as *tidal breaths*. How does your respiration rate compare with that of your classmate(s)?

   (Normal adult respiratory rate range is 14-20 breaths per minute.)

II. **The effect of body position and tension on maximum phonation duration (MPD)**

   A. The task of maximum phonation duration uses vital capacity (maximum inspiration followed by maximum expiration) coupled with vocal fold vibration. Practice this task by taking a deep breath and sustaining /*a*/ (as in "odd") at a comfortable pitch and loudness level until you have no more air.

   Record your time: _____ (MPD varies with age, gender, stature, physical condition, and experience with the task.)

   B. Perform two trials of MPD for /a/ for each of the following postures†: Have your partner record your times.

	Trial 1	Trial 2
1. Standing straight	_____	_____
2. Lying supine	_____	_____
3. Sitting straight	_____	_____
4. Sitting slouched	_____	_____
5. Maximally tensing torso	_____	_____

   †Rest between trials

   C. From **your** data, what observations can you make?

   D. What clinical implications do posture and tension have on respiration and phonation?

   E. Aerodynamic measures of airflow rate and air pressure are more informative than MPD. Read about these measures and their manner of assessment.

   1. With a space-occupying lesion or vocal fold paralysis in which glottal closure is incomplete, would MPD be **increased** or **decreased**? Would airflow rate be **increased** or **decreased**? Would air pressure at the glottis be **increased** or **decreased**? (*Circle the correct answers.*)

   2. With adductor spasmodic dysphonia in which glottal closure is tight, would MPD be **increased** or **decreased**? Would airflow rate be **increased** or **decreased**? Would air pressure at the glottis be **increased** or **decreased**? (*Circle the correct answers.*)

III. **S/Z ratio**

   A. The task of sustaining and comparing maximum sustained /s/ with /z/, allows the clinician to compare respiratory function *without* vocal fold vibration (/s/) to that *with* vocal fold vibration (/z/). Contrasting /s/ and /z/ strives to reduce airflow and air pressure variability within the vocal tract above the glottis.

   B. Taking a deep breath, sustain /s/ (sound a snake makes) until all of your air is expended. Time and then record two trials of /s/. _____ _____

Copyright © 2007 by Mosby, Inc., an affiliate of Elsevier Inc. All rights reserved.

C. Taking a deep breath, sustain /z/ (sound a bee makes) until all of your air is expended. Time and then record two trials of /z/. _____ _____

D. Determine your S/Z ratio by dividing the longest /s/ time by the longest /z/ time (s/z) Record your quotient: _____

E. Your quotient should approximate 1.0 if your vocal folds are fully closing. Would you expect someone with unilateral vocal fold paralysis (one vocal fold doesn't close) to have an S/Z ratio that is greater or less than 1.0? Explain your answer.

F. What can the clinician infer when the S/Z ratio exceeds 1.0? Eckel and Boone[21] found that 90% of the subjects in their study who had nodules and polyps had S/Z ratios in excess of 1.4. Based on their findings, can the clinician presume that the client has a space-occupying lesion based on their S/Z ratio? Why or why not?

IV. **Respiration for speech**

A. Read the "Rainbow Passage" (Fairbanks, 1960 [see p. 111]) to a partner or tape record it. Time the reading. It contains 100 words. Place a mark wherever a breath is taken. Determine how many breaths were taken.
Record here: _____ breaths _____ total seconds required to read

B. Divide the total time required for reading by the number of breaths to determine the average number of seconds per breath. (*Example*: If the passage was read in 42 seconds with 7 breaths, the average number of seconds per breath is 6 seconds.)
Record here: _____ average seconds per breath
Daniloff, Schucker, and Feth[20] noted that at conversational loudness levels, normal phrasing is 2.4-3.5 seconds per phrase.

C. How does that time compare with your MPD for /a/? What can you conclude?

D. Did your classmate(s) take breaths at the same places in the passage that you did?

E. What does this suggest about respiration and phrasing when reading aloud? Is it true for speech also?

F. Divide the total number of words in the passage (100) by the number of breaths that you took to determine the number of words per breath. (*Example*: 100 words read in 6 breaths; mean words per breath would be 17.)
Record here: _____ words per breath

G. If one's vocal cords did not close completely, as in the case of vocal cord paralysis, would that person take more or less breaths when talking? How would that coincide with the number of words per breath? Explain your answer.

V. **Remediation Research and Discussion Questions**

1. What medical professions are concerned with assessment and treatment of respiratory problems?

2. What instrumentation is used to measure respiratory volumes, flows, and pressures? What are the units of measurement?

3. What is pulse oximetry? How is it measured? What percentage is considered within normal limits?

4. Discuss clinical situations in which it is appropriate for the speech-language pathologist to work with a client's breathing.

5. The terms *clavicular breathing* and *breathing from the diaphragm* are often seen in texts and espoused by professional voice users. Explain these terms. Under what conditions are these breathing methods used?

---

*References 4, 10, 15, 17, 21, 24, 33-35, 53.

Copyright © 2007 by Mosby, Inc., an affiliate of Elsevier Inc. All rights reserved.

VOICE ANALYSIS LAB*

ASHA CERTIFICATION STANDARDS ADDRESSED: III-B, III-C, III-D, IV-B

MATERIALS NEEDED: CAPE-V sentences and rating form; "Rainbow Passage" (see page 111) Pitch analysis instrument; musical scale with Hz conversion (see page 113) Voice Handicap Index (see page 118); voice norms (see page 114) Tape recorder; watch with second hand

Name: _____ Partner: _____ Date: _____

PITCH

1. Habitual pitch—CAPE-V rating: Low____ High____ Appropriate____
2. Speaking fundamental frequency (SFF): Instrument used: _____
   Sustained /a/_____Hz   Contextual speech (counting) _____Hz
   Is this within normal limits for age and sex? _____
3. Fundamental frequency phonation (pitch) range

   ### Instructions:

   ■ "Start at a comfortable pitch level and go as high as you can using an /a/ sound."
   ■ "Start at a comfortable pitch level and go as low as you can using an /a/ sound."
      You may imitate a siren, or sing notes on a scale.
      Siren Up   maximum Hz _____   Siren Down   minimum Hz
      Scale Up   maximum Hz _____   Scale Down   minimum Hz
   ■ Using the highest and the lowest numbers recorded above, determine the following:
      Whole tones (white piano keys) within your range _____
      Semitones (white and black keys) within your range _____
      Is your range within normal limits? _____
4. Frequency perturbation (jitter) for /a/ _____
   Is your perturbation within normal limits?_____
   Instrument used: _____
   Explain frequency and intensity perturbation to your partner. Perceptually when the client has a large perturbation value, how might he or she sound?

QUALITY

1. Using the CAPE-V protocol, with percentages or a 0 to 5 severity scale, listen to the voice and rate the following:
   Overall severity____ Roughness____ Breathiness____ Strain____ Glottal fry_____
   Glottal attacks____ Phonation breaks____ Aphonia____ Other____
   0 = normal; 1 = mild; 2 = mild-moderate; 3 = moderate; 4 = moderate-severe; 5 = severe
2. Acoustical analysis of voice quality:
   Using instrumentation that measures signal complexity, follow the instructions to accurately measure the voice signal.
   Instrument used:

   _____

   What it measured:

   _____

   Findings:

   _____

   Do your acoustic findings "match" your perceptual findings?

Copyright © 2007 by Mosby, Inc., an affiliate of Elsevier Inc. All rights reserved.

LOUDNESS

1. Habitual loudness—CAPE-V rating: Quiet_____ Loud_____ Appropriate_____
2. Habitual (mean) intensity /a/_____dB. Is this within normal limits? _____
Instrument used: _____
What contrasts do you notice between hertz (Hz) and decibels (dB)?
When measuring the intensity of one's voice, why is mouth to microphone distance so important?

RESPIRATION

1. Observe your partner's nonspeech breathing. Where do you see movement?
2. MPD for /a/ _____sec Is this within normal limits? _____
3. S/Z RATIO /s/____ sec /z/____ sec Ratio_____ Is this within normal limits? ____

VOCAL ABUSE RATING

0 = never; 1 = seldom; 2 = sometimes; 3 = often; 4 = very often; 5 = always
_____ Shouting/yelling/screaming
_____ Talking loudly
_____ Talking over noise
_____ Phone use
_____ Singing
_____ Making noises/using different voices
_____ Coughing/throat clearing

VOICE HANDICAP INDEX

TOTAL SCORE _____/120
Physical impact _____/40
Functional impact _____/40
Emotional impact _____/40

RATE

Appropriate _____ Excessive _____ Slow _____
Words per minute—reading rate: _____

LARYNGEAL PALPATION

1. _____ Locate the hyoid bone
2. _____ Locate the thyroid cartilage
3. _____ Locate the thyrohyoid space
Pretending that your partner is an actual client; summarize the findings from your "evaluation," and provide appropriate recommendations.

REMEDIATION RESEARCH AND DISCUSSION QUESTIONS

1. Discuss when a laryngeal examination is indicated for a client/patient who presents with a voice disorder. (Refer to the "ASHA Preferred Practice Patterns" in this text [see page 89].)
2. Discuss the advantages and disadvantages of each method of laryngeal examination.
Indirect mirror examination:
Flexible nasoendoscopy:
Rigid oral laryngoscopy:
Stroboscopy:
3. What knowledge and skills are needed by the speech-language pathologist (SLP) performing laryngeal imaging? Can he or she diagnose laryngeal pathology?
4. Why can't the SLP use acoustic, perceptual, aerodynamic or electroglottography measures to diagnose vocal pathology? What is the utility of these measures?

---

*References 4, 8-11, 15, 17, 21, 24, 53, 56, 61, 66, 67.

Copyright © 2007 by Mosby, Inc., an affiliate of Elsevier Inc. All rights reserved.

ASHA CERTIFICATION STANDARDS ADDRESSED: III-B, III-C, III-D

MATERIALS NEEDED: gloves, flashlight, tongue depressor, small mirror, diagram† of oral cavity and nasopharynx

Name: _____ Partner: _____ Date: _____

I. **Observe the following oral structures and note any deviances:**
   A. Height of the palate, appearance of palate and uvula, presence of tonsils
   B. Dentition, occlusion
   C. Where are the adenoids located? Can they be seen in an oral examination?

II. **Perform the following assessments:**
   A. Have your "client" sustain "ah;" observe velum for movement and symmetry. Can velopharyngeal closure be seen?
   B. Trigger a gag reflex. At which anatomical location was it triggered?

III. **Assess and learn about nasal resonance by having the client do the following:**
   A. Close his or her mouth; observe nasal breathing. Note and explain any abnormality.
   B. Observe the structure of the nose. Note any deviance.
   C. Have the client sustain /n/, /m/, /ŋ/ with a mirror held below the nose and above the mouth.
   What do you observe?
   D. Say /n/, /m/, /ŋ/ while placing your thumb and index finger on the sides of the nose. What do you feel?
   E. Sustain /a/, /i/, /u/ with a mirror below the nose and above the mouth. What do you observe?
   F. Say theses sentences in a normal tone of voice.
   My name means money. Susie sews zippers for Sherry.
   Use the "mirror" and the "thumb-finger" test. What do you observe?
   G. Sustain /z/ and /s/ with audible nasal emission holding the mirror in the same position.
   (Nasal emission is created by forcing air up through the nasopharynx to produce an outward snort sound.) What do you observe and feel?
   H. Say the sentences in (F) with **excessive** nasality. Use the "mirror" and the "thumb-finger" test. What do you observe?
   I. Would nasal or non-nasal consonants provide the best information for diagnosing hypernasality? Explain.
   J. Produce the following sound substitutions and describe how they are produced:
   - Nasal emission on /s/
   - Glottal stop (by making the sound in the middle of "uh oh")
   K. Why would someone with velopharyngeal incompetence have these sound substitutions as part of their deviant speech pattern?

IV. **Assess and learn about hyponasality.**
   A. Say this sentence without letting any air flow through your nose.
   We need meaning men.
   B. The denasal substitution for /n/ is ___; /m/ is ___; /ŋ/ is ___.
   C. Using the "mirror" and "thumb-finger" tests, repeat the task in section A above. What do you notice?

V. **Task to differentiate hypernasality from hyponasality.**
   A. Say these sentences, first with nares open; then with nares occluded.
   My nanny knows no one. Mary makes more money.

---

† Included in this book.

Copyright © 2007 by Mosby, Inc., an affiliate of Elsevier Inc. All rights reserved.

■ If the client is hypernasal, will there be a perceptual difference between these two conditions? Why or why not?

■ If the client is hyponasal, will there be a perceptual difference between these two conditions? Why or why not?

VI. Remediation research and discussion questions:

A. Do oral motor activities help remediate hypernasality?

B. Can nasality and nasal emission be phonological process errors in a person with normal resonance?

C. Once hypernasality or hyponasality is detected through simple clinical tests, what additional diagnostic steps should be taken?

D. What commercial products and instruments are available for acoustic and aerodynamic assessment of nasal resonance?

E. What types of professions are represented on a cleft palate team?

---

*References 4, 9, 10, 15, 27, 38.

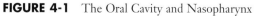

FIGURE 4-1 The Oral Cavity and Nasopharynx

Copyright © 2007 by Mosby, Inc., an affiliate of Elsevier Inc. All rights reserved.

ALARYNGEAL SPEECH LAB*

ASHA STANDARDS ADDRESSED: III-B, III-C, III-D

MATERIALS NEEDED: Electrolarynges; diagrams of prelaryngectomy and postlaryngectomy†; computer with internet access; alcohol wipes

Helpful websites: • *www.luminaud.com* • *www.larynxlink.com* • *www.griffinlab.com* • *www.brucemedical.com* • *www.inhealth.com*

Name: _____ Partner(s): _____ Date: _____

I. **Anatomical and physiological changes caused by a laryngectomy**
   A. Explain to your "patient" (partner) who will undergo a total laryngectomy the anatomical and physiological changes that he will experience. Use diagrams.
   Breathing
   Talking
   Hygiene
   Eating
   B. Discuss with your client the various professionals who will comprise the treatment team and what the speech-language pathologist's (SLP's) role will be.

II. **Speech options following laryngectomy—tracheoesophageal puncture**
   A. Your patient will be having a tracheoesophageal puncture (TEP) procedure at the time of the laryngectomy. Discuss this procedure, and how it will allow them to speak.
   B. Discuss with your patient methods he or she can use to communicate during the initial postoperative period, before the T-E voice is usable.

III. **Speech options following laryngectomy—electrolarynges****
   A. What is the name of the electrolarynx that you are using?
   B. Is it a neck or an intraoral device?
   C. If it is a neck device, can it be converted to an intraoral device? What would be the benefit of this?
   D. Does your electrolarynx use disposable or rechargeable batteries?
   E. Can it be adjusted for loudness?
   F. Can it be adjusted for pitch?
   G. How many hands are required to operate the electrolarynx? If more than one hand, how is this a disadvantage?
   H. Using the electrolarynx, experiment with your partner to find the optimal placement for understandable speech. How would you aid your client in consistently locating his or her optimal placement?
   I. Practice saying the following:
      ▪ Sustained vowels
      ▪ Counting to 20; saying the alphabet, days of the week, months
      ▪ Novel words, phrases, sentences
      Is the speaker understandable? How did each of you feel when speech was not understandable?
   J. Using an electrolarynx, find a listener unfamiliar with the speech aid, and ask them a question or engage them in conversation. Discuss the listener's response and how you felt using the device.
   K. Research: What is the initial cost of your electrolarynx? What will be the ongoing cost? Is it covered by Medicare? Does it have a warranty? What is the name of the website that you used?

---

†Included in this book.

**Take turns using the device within your group, then switch electrolarynges with another group and repeat activities in section III.

Copyright © 2007 by Mosby, Inc., an affiliate of Elsevier Inc. All rights reserved.

IV. **Speech options following laryngectomy—esophageal speech**
   A. Discuss with your "patient" (partner) how esophageal speech is produced. Describe the mechanism and methods whereby air is trapped in the esophagus.
   Consonant injection
   Prephonation
   Inhalation
   B. With your partner, attempt each of the air intake methods below. (If you can voluntarily belch, what method is used to trap the air?) Were you successful at putting in air? How do you know? What method did you use?
      1. Consonant injection: Use words such as *post, toast, chop, coke.*
      2. Prephonation: Trap the air by pressing your lips together; or your tongue against your alveolar ridge; or against your soft palate.
      3. Inhalation: Quickly sniff in the air with an "open" throat.
   C. After trapping air, can sound be produced?
      ■ Say /a/ as in "odd."
      ■ Try changing the sound to a different vowel.
      ■ Try saying a single-syllable word.
      ■ Try saying your name.
   D. How do you feel (physically) after practicing esophageal speech?
   E. What is your psychological reaction to the sound of esophageal speech?
V. **Remediation research and discussion questions**
   A. If a patient asks if one method of alaryngeal speech is better than another, how would you answer?
   B. Should the speech-language pathologist be allowed to fit, place, and replace the T-E puncture prosthesis? What training should be required before doing this? (Check out ASHA Position Statements, Supplement 24, 2004.)
   C. If the speech-language pathologist is unable to personally achieve voice with esophageal speech, is she/he credible to teach it to a laryngectomized patient?
   D. Under what conditions would someone be a poor candidate for a T-E puncture?
   E. What are some of the psychosocial issues that having a laryngectomy might create? How can these issues be addressed?

---

*References 1, 2, 4, 7, 8, 16, 18, 19.

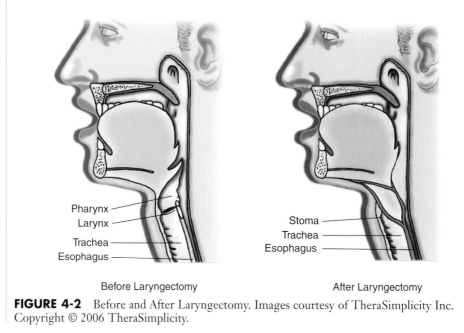

Pharynx
Larynx
Trachea
Esophagus

Stoma
Trachea
Esophagus

Before Laryngectomy   After Laryngectomy

FIGURE 4-2   Before and After Laryngectomy. Images courtesy of TheraSimplicity Inc. Copyright © 2006 TheraSimplicity.

Copyright © 2007 by Mosby, Inc., an affiliate of Elsevier Inc. All rights reserved.

"Unsolved" Case Studies

Ten incomplete case studies are presented, five pediatric/adolescent and five adult, representing a range of voice disorders. **If the disorder did not appear in the previous case studies, an explanation of it is given preceding the case study.** For example, paralysis was discussed in the first section of the book, so readers should turn to the page number provided to re-read the explanation. Recurrent respiratory papilloma (RRP) did not appear in a previous case study, thus the explanation is found just before the unsolved case study on RRP.

Before delving into the unsolved cases, a solved case study is provided to serve as a guide for clinical thinking and problem solving. Using the guided example, the student can read each section of the diagnostic report and then check to see whether his or her analysis and synthesis of the information matches that which is in italics.

Solving the case studies requires listening to the voice samples; identifying pertinent medical, voice, developmental, and social/emotional information; interpreting the evaluation findings, choosing appropriate trial therapy techniques, and summarizing the findings; making appropriate recommendations; and determining treatment goals. In addition to the guided learning sample, students are encouraged to review the case studies in the first section of the book. Gaining "hands on" experience with the diagnostic process will greatly increase the student's knowledge, skills, and comfort with voice and laryngeal disorders.

Copyright © 2007 by Mosby, Inc., an affiliate of Elsevier Inc. All rights reserved.

UNSOLVED CASE STUDY

GUIDED LEARNING EXAMPLE: MUSCLE TENSION DYSPHONIA

Voice clip #21

See page **18** for overview.

BACKGROUND AND REASONS FOR REFERRAL

Richie, a 7-year-old male about to enter second grade, was seen for a voice evaluation. He was accompanied by his mother. The presenting complaint was vocal hoarseness that has been present for several years.

HISTORY

According to the client's mother, Richie has been receiving speech and language therapy since age 2 for a developmental speech and language delay. Secondarily, vocal hoarseness has been noted. Richie has been examined twice by an otolaryngologist, once through indirect laryngoscopy with a mirror and subsequently with a flexible nasolaryngoscope. Neither examination has revealed any structural abnormalities of the larynx or vocal folds. Both folds are noted to move fully and symmetrically, with signs of increased laryngeal tension during phonation. Voice therapy has been a part of his overall speech and language therapy, but according to his school speech-language pathologist (SLP), Richie's voice has not improved. This evaluation was requested by the school SLP to provide additional diagnostic information and voice therapy ideas and resources for this client.

Mother reported that Richie has sounded hoarse for as long as she remembers. She does not observe changes in his voice quality coinciding with allergy season. She does note that his voice fatigues with continued use as the day progresses. Richie likes to make "guttural sounds" when he plays, but she feels that Richie's voice use is no different from that of her other sons.

Richie has had frequent ear infections. He did not have colic as a baby. He has had no surgeries or injuries involving the head or neck. He does not have allergies or asthma. His fluid intake is good. He takes no medications regularly. Richie receives tutoring for reading. He receives occupational therapy (OT) for improvement of fine motor coordination and oral motor skills. According to Richie's mother, his voice currently is not affecting him negatively with regard to academic performance or social interactions. She feels, however, that an eventual negative impact will be experienced.

Clinical Thinking: History

1. What questions need to be answered?
   a. If this problem is functional muscle tension dysphonia (MTD)[61] what is causing it?
   b. Why have previous therapy attempts been unsuccessful?
   c. What new information, insight, treatment ideas, or recommendations can I bring to this case?
2. From this history, what information is significant for a voice problem?
   a. Possibly the speech and language delay. Could a great desire to communicate result in excessive laryngeal muscle tension and effort?
   b. Frequent ear infections. Is he speaking too loudly, resulting in increased vocal effort?
   c. Several active boy siblings in the family. Is the problem the result of vocal abuse?
   d. OT and SLP for motor coordination problems. Do these problems carry over into phonation?

Copyright © 2007 by Mosby, Inc., an affiliate of Elsevier Inc. All rights reserved.

3. What can be ruled out (although the clinician should always be watchful for inaccurate information)?
    a. Laryngeal pathology, congenital or acquired
    b. Allergies, reflux, negative medication effects
    c. Inadequate hydration
4. What additional questions would I like to ask the referring SLP, parent, or child?
    a. Example: In what sports does this child participate? How frequently does he play? How involved does he get in the sport? How does he use his voice during the practices and games?
    b. When was the last time his larynx was examined? What was the method? May I have a copy of the report or directly contact the physician?
5. How severe is the problem and what is its impact on the client and family?
    a. It is not currently impacting the child socially, emotionally, physically, or academically.
    b. Mom is concerned that there will be a negative impact as he matures.

EVALUATION
Pitch

Speaking fundamental frequency for sustained /a/ was 283 Hz. Habitual pitch for contextual speech was 269 Hz, *which is within normal limits for his age and gender.*[17] A phonation range from 206-719 Hz, 13 whole tones, was elicited with a phonation break at 518 Hz. *(Adult phonation ranges typically surpass 16 whole tones or 25 semitones.[17])* Frequency perturbation for /a/ was 1.16%. *(Normal voices are typically associated with a frequency perturbation that is less than 1%.[53])*

Quality

Breathiness was rated as 3 (moderate), roughness as 2 (mild to moderate), and vocal strain as 3 (moderate). Phonation breaks, hard glottal attacks, and intermittent difficulty with phonation onset were present. Dysphonia was consistent throughout the evaluation.

Loudness

Modal loudness for /a/ was 72 dB. Perceptually loudness was within normal limits for a quiet environment.

Respiration

Maximum phonation duration for /a/ was 10 seconds, *which is within normal limits.*[17] S/Z ratio was 1.2 (10 and 8 seconds, respectively), *which exceeds normal limits.*[70] Normal breathing patterns were observed.

Musculoskeletal Tension

Excessive laryngeal strap muscle use was observed during phonation, particularly in the sternocleidomastoids. Following laryngeal massage,[11] there appeared to be a small improvement in voice quality.

Vocal Abuse Behaviors

The following behaviors were identified and rated on a 0 to 5 scale (5 most frequently occurring):
    4—Shouting, yelling, screaming
    3—Talking in the presence of competing noise
    3—Making loud, harsh noises
    3—Overall amount of talking

Copyright © 2007 by Mosby, Inc., an affiliate of Elsevier Inc. All rights reserved.

Articulation

Developmental articulation errors heard on /l/, /r/, /ð/ and /θ/.

Clinical Thinking: Evaluation

1. For each voice area, are the diagnostic results within normal limits?
   a. Is habitual pitch within normal limits for his age and sex?
   b. Does the pitch of /a/ match that of contextual speech? If no, how discrepant are they?
   c. Perceptually, do I agree with the acoustic results?
   d. As I listen to his voice quality, what would I imagine vocal fold vibration and closure to look like?
   e. What does the discrepancy between /s/ and /z/ indicate?
2. If the diagnostic results are not within normal limits, what does that suggest?
   a. Musculoskeletal tension assessment suggests increased laryngeal tension.
   b. The consistency of the voice quality suggests most probably a gradual onset disorder and quality that is not amenable to dramatic change during trial therapy.
   c. These will be the areas to target in therapy, or the areas to continually assess as determinants of progress.

TRIAL THERAPY

At the conclusion of the evaluation, the voice technique of "confidential voice" was taught to Richie and his mother. It was explained that confidential voice could be used in many different speaking situations and would help to reduce laryngeal hyperfunction. Richie practiced first using confidential voice while doing rote tasks such as counting. He then practiced it while doing a picture description activity and playing a card game. Laryngeal massage was not taught to the client during the initial evaluation because it was felt that he was too young to independently perform this technique. Additionally, one vocal abuse behavior was chosen to target its reduction throughout the upcoming week, with suggestions provided for substituting nonvocally abusive behaviors in its place.

Clinical Thinking: Trial Therapy

1. Are there any therapy techniques that will make an immediate improvement in his voice? Possibly laryngeal massage11 might make a difference.
2. Are there any techniques that can be initiated at the time of the evaluation that can be worked on during the interim until the next therapy appointment? Possibly confidential voice17 might help.
3. Is education of voice abuse, misuse, vocal hygiene, and daily charting the best starting point? This is a good starting point but hasn't it already been targeted in previous therapy sessions?

SUMMARY

This 7-year-old male presents with a voice disorder characterized by breathiness, roughness, and strain. Though voice has sounded like this for several years, according to otolaryngology report, there is no evidence of a structural abnormality of the larynx or vocal folds. Thus he appears to have a muscle tension dysphonia.

During today's evaluation, several observations were made that might explain the etiology of Richie's dysphonia. Richie's conversation reveals an effortful or deliberate process at three levels: language encoding, articulation, and phonation. Possibly, this voice disorder is the result of initially misusing and abusing his voice when trying to communicate with reduced verbal language skills, which has become a habitual way of phonating for him. He appears to "try hard" at all levels when communicating. He also demonstrated some "play noises" that he uses (with less frequency now, according to his mother) that were extremely vocally abusive. Finally, he was observed to snort frequently throughout the session, and his mother

Copyright © 2007 by Mosby, Inc., an affiliate of Elsevier Inc. All rights reserved.

NOTES

commented on his frequent burping, both possibly indicating a laryngopharyngeal reflux (LPR) component.

Clinical Thinking: Summary

1. Summarize all significant findings in a succinct but accurate and complete manner. (Someone receiving this report may take the time to read only the summary section.)
2. Given the information from this diagnostic, what do you believe is the voice diagnosis?
3. Can you hypothesize, based on information gathered, the cause (etiology) of the problem?

RECOMMENDATIONS

1. To continue voice therapy as part of his overall speech and language treatment plan.
2. To monitor and reduce voice misuse and abuse in the home, school, and play environments, substituting nonvocal behaviors whenever possible.
3. To discuss reflux indications and trial medical management with the otolaryngologist.
4. To reduce vocal effort through laryngeal massage and voice facilitative techniques such as yawn sigh, confidential voice, and reduced loudness.
5. To undergo laryngeal stroboscopy to rule out subtle vocal fold pathology if voice quality is unchanged despite family compliance.

Clinical Thinking: Recommendations

What recommendations are appropriate and indicated?
    a. Is voice therapy recommended? With what frequency and projected length?
    b. How will the therapy differ from what has currently been tried?
    c. Is further medical information and evaluation needed?
    d. Are ancillary services indicated?
    e. Is family and teacher education needed?

Long-term Treatment Goals

Richie will reduce the negative voice characteristics of MTD through using appropriate facilitative techniques, reducing vocal abuse, and improving vocal hygiene, as assessed through perceptual ratings of 2 (mild to moderate) or less and relative average perturbation within the normal range.

Clinical Thinking: Long-term Treatment Goals

1. What would be a realistic successful therapy outcome for this client?
2. Can a return of "normal" voice be anticipated?

Short-term Treatment Goals

1. Richie will learn about voice structure and function and healthy voice choices as assessed after testing, earning a score of 75% or more.
2. Richie will reduce vocal strain by using yawn sigh,[15] confidential voice,[17] and laryngeal massage[11] techniques as assessed through clinician and client effort ratings of less than 2 on a 0-3 effort rating scale.
3. Richie will reduce his frequency of vocal abuse behaviors by using substitute nonvocal behaviors and self-control, as assessed through posttreatment vocal abuse ratings demonstrating a reduction of minimally 1 point.

Clinical Thinking: Short-term Treatment Goals

1. What sub-goals will allow the long-term treatment goal to be met?
2. How will they be assessed?
3. Are they realistic?
4. Can they be further subdivided to form objectives for each therapy session?

Copyright © 2007 by Mosby, Inc., an affiliate of Elsevier Inc. All rights reserved.

"Unsolved" Case Studies: Pediatric

RECURRENT RESPIRATORY PAPILLOMATOSIS

 Voice clip #22

OVERVIEW

Recurrent respiratory papillomatosis (RRP), also known as *papilloma*, involves wartlike benign growths that occur in the larynx, trachea, and other structures of the upper aerodigestive tract. The disease is viral based, being associated with the human papillomavirus (HPV). It is a disease first experienced in early childhood and can be life long, but is often reported to abate at puberty. It arises from the epithelium, and when on the vocal folds, it typically causes hoarseness. When it proliferates, it can invade the airway causing breathing problems. As its name implies, it recurs after no set time interval, requiring the patient to have a long-term relationship with the otolaryngologist. Medical and surgical options are used ranging from interferon injections to forceps and laser surgical removal.

The occurrence of RRP is relatively rare: 4.3 cases per 100,000 children reported by Verdolini, Rosen, and Branski (2006).[73] Because of its serious nature, however, children with hoarseness or breathing compromise not attributable to acute or chronic respiratory conditions, should have laryngeal examinations. The SLP cannot diagnose the cause of hoarseness based on perceptual voice characteristics.

The speech-language pathologist's role varies with each client with RRP. For the pediatric client who has never been diagnosed with RRP and is severely hoarse, breathy, and strained, with possible respiratory compromise, the SLP's role is that of identification and immediate referral for medical diagnosis and treatment. For the client who has already been diagnosed with RRP, the SLP's role is to monitor the client's voice and be watchful for changes that might indicate recurrence of papilloma. Additional goals are helping the patients establish his or her best voice while educating the client on vocal abuse, vocal hygiene, reduced vocal hyperfunction and assisting the client in developing tolerance for ongoing laryngeal imaging and surgery.

The "unsolved" case study of Marietta is included to acquaint the SLP with the challenges unique to the client with RRP. At the time that Marietta presented for voice therapy, she had undergone only one surgery for removal of papilloma, yet her voice was significantly disordered. This was due to the extent of surgical intervention, as well as the muscle tension dysphonia phonation pattern that had been established before surgery. It is hoped that as the SLP researches this case, an appreciation for the challenge that RRP poses will be gained and the value of voice therapy, medical and surgical intervention and management, and counseling for these clients and their families will be recognized.

BACKGROUND AND REASONS FOR REFERRAL

Marietta, a 4-year-old female with a prior history of RRP of the larynx, was seen for a voice evaluation. According to Marietta's mother, the presenting complaint is failure to regain normal voice after surgical removal of papilloma, which occurred 5 weeks before this evaluation.

HISTORY

According to parent report, Marietta was adopted at birth. Little was known about her prenatal care or biological family history. Approximately 5 months ago, a gradual onset of hoarseness that increased in severity was noted. Marietta's parents also had

Copyright © 2007 by Mosby, Inc., an affiliate of Elsevier Inc. All rights reserved.

noted a stridorous noise accompanying her breathing during strenuous play. Marietta was seen by her pediatrician and prescribed antibiotics, which did not produce a change. Marietta was then referred to a pediatric otolaryngologist. Her larynx was examined through flexible nasoendoscopy. She was diagnosed with papilloma of the vocal folds and subglottis. The papilloma was surgically removed by laser. She did not require a tracheotomy. The family was counseled on the serious and recurring nature of papilloma. Follow-up voice therapy was recommended, but not initially pursued.

According to Marietta's mother, Marietta eats and sleeps well. She is in good health. Other than vitamins, no medications are taken regularly. She enjoys preschool; however, her teacher notes that since surgery she speaks much less than previously, preferring to make her needs known through noises and gestures.

OBSERVATIONS

Marietta used a combination of whisper and effortful phonation for the majority of her speech attempts but was intermittently noted to phonate on inhalation. Her attention span was very limited, moving rapidly from one activity to another. Voice data was gathered through audio recordings during play because she would not cooperate for an acoustic analysis.

EVALUATION
Pitch

Fundamental frequency for supraglottic sounding phonation was 191-219 Hz, which is significantly low for her age. Fundamental frequency range (measured as Marietta imitated a siren while phonating on inhalation) was 340-720 Hz, which is approximately nine whole notes. Frequency perturbation was not measured.

Quality

Quality ranged from intermittent whispering to effortful supraglottic phonation. A normal sounding voice quality was heard on inhalation. She was observed to use inhalation phonation when making play noises or when wanting her mother's attention. Her laugh was without phonation.

Loudness

Perceptually judged as reduced when whispering or using effortful phonation; within normal limits to excessive when phonating on inhalation.

Respiration

Normal breathing patterns observed at rest without effort or stridor. Whisper accompanied both inhalation and exhalation. Maximum phonation duration for /a/ (produced on inhalation) was 8 seconds and did not appear to reach her maximum capability.

Vocal Abuse Behaviors

Supraglottic phonation
Whisper phonation
Inhalation phonation

Resonation
Within normal limits.

Articulation
Developmental articulation errors noted.

Language
Functionally appropriate, but was not formally assessed.

Copyright © 2007 by Mosby, Inc., an affiliate of Elsevier Inc. All rights reserved.

TRIAL THERAPY

SUMMARY

RECOMMENDATIONS

Long-term Treatment Goals

Short-term Treatment Goals

Copyright © 2007 by Mosby, Inc., an affiliate of Elsevier Inc. All rights reserved.

NOTES

UNSOLVED CASE STUDY 2

VOCAL NODULES

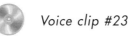 *Voice clip #23*

See page **36** for overview.

BACKGROUND AND REASONS FOR REFERRAL

Rachael is a 2-year, 5-month-old female who was seen for a voice evaluation, secondary to a diagnosis of bilateral vocal nodules. The presenting complaints include vocal roughness and voice loss after crying. Rachael was accompanied by her mother.

HISTORY

According to Rachael's mother, Rachael's birth and developmental history were medically unremarkable. Rachael's speech and language development was reported as single words at 10 months, two-word phrases at 15 months, and talking in sentences at 19 months.

It was reported by Rachael's mother that as a baby she presented with a normal cry. Hoarseness occurred gradually, between 15 to 18 months of age. Eventually, Rachael began losing her voice after temper tantrums. Currently Rachael is reported to yell, talk loudly, and speak excessively "much of the time," which according to her mother, is thought to be the cause of her voice problem. Voice quality is hoarse most of the time, worsening after periods of crying. Rachael is in preschool two mornings per week, including music class 1 hour per week.

Rachael is not exposed to smoke. She presents with seasonal allergy symptoms but is not currently taking medication. There is no report of laryngopharyngeal reflux symptoms. Rachael's fluid intake consists of roughly three glasses per day. She is currently undergoing toilet training, thus her mother is trying to limit fluids. Their home has a central humidifier. Rachael is an only child, living with both parents.

OBSERVATIONS

Rachael presented as observant and interested in her surroundings. She attempted all presented speech tasks with occasional coaxing from her mother. She enjoyed conversing with the clinician. She attended to each activity for approximately 5 minutes.

EVALUATION
Pitch

Speaking fundamental frequency for /a/ was 328 Hz, and for contextual speech 314 Hz. Phonation range was not measured because of client's difficulty with the task. When singing "Happy Birthday," phonation breaks were heard on higher notes. Pitch inflections were within normal limits.

Quality

Overall voice severity was rated as 4 (moderate to severe). Breathiness was rated as 3 (moderate), roughness was rated as 2 (mild to moderate), and strain was rated as 4 (moderate to severe). Voice was not breathy. Phonation breaks and hard glottal attacks were heard.

Loudness

Voice was inappropriately loud for the treatment room. This coincides with observations made by her mother.

Respiration

Normal breathing patterns observed.

Copyright © 2007 by Mosby, Inc., an affiliate of Elsevier Inc. All rights reserved.

Vocal Abuse Behaviors

The following behaviors were rated by Rachael's mother on a 0 to 5 scale with 5 representing behaviors that are most frequent or severe:

3—Shouting, yelling, screaming
3—Talking in the presence of noise
3—Singing loudly
4—Talking excessively
5—Talking loudly

Resonation

Within normal limits; mild hyponasality was heard.

Articulation

Age appropriate.

Rate

Within normal limits.

Language

Above normal limits for her age.

Hearing

Tested at 6 months of age and found to be within normal limits.

Copyright © 2007 by Mosby, Inc., an affiliate of Elsevier Inc. All rights reserved.

TRIAL THERAPY

SUMMARY

RECOMMENDATIONS

Long-term Treatment Goals

Short-term Treatment Goals

Copyright © 2007 by Mosby, Inc., an affiliate of Elsevier Inc. All rights reserved.

UNSOLVED CASE STUDY 3

STATUS FOLLOWING PHARYNGEAL FLAP REPAIR FOR CLEFT PALATE

 Voice clip #24

See page **79** for overview.

BACKGROUND AND REASONS FOR REFERRAL

Ashley is a 6-year-old home-schooled female. She presented with voice, resonance, and articulation problems secondary to a cleft lip and palate that have both been repaired, the latter through pharyngeal flap surgery. She is monitored by a craniofacial team at a reputable medical center but has not had ongoing speech therapy. Indirect mirror laryngoscopy revealed bilateral vocal fold thickening at the anterior third, posterior two-thirds juncture.

EVALUATION
Oral Peripheral Evaluation

LIPS   A scar was observed in the center of the upper lip as a result of a repaired cleft lip. The upper lip was short and slightly raised at midline. The bottom lip appeared normal. Lips were symmetrical and are closed at rest. During speech productions, both upper and lower lips were retracted.

DENTITION   The client presented with a class III malocclusion[53] (i.e., the mandible protruded forward beyond her maxilla). Diastemas (spaces between teeth) were present, especially between the teeth of the maxilla arch. Malpositioned teeth on the maxillary arch were observed.

TONGUE   The tongue appeared normal in size and tone. Tongue resting position was at the front of her mouth, near her front teeth.

Respiration

Air exchange was primarily through her mouth, rather than her nose. Audible mouth breathing was observed.

Resonation

Resonance and voice were evaluated through an informal play format with audio recording. Ashley's resonance during speech tasks evidenced significant denasality (reduced nasal resonance), presumably resulting from the pharyngeal flap. Perceptually /n/, /m/, and /ŋ/ phonemes resembled /d/, /b/, and /g/ (respectively). On sustained vowels, however, mild hypernasality was heard. No nasal emission was noted.

Articulation

Overall intelligibility was affected by multiple articulation errors. Intermittently glottal stops were substituted for plosives and affricates.

Rate

Rapid, with minimal mouth and articulator excursion when speaking.

Voice

Moderate hoarseness and increased vocal effort were noted, most likely caused by her compensatory use of increased effort to close the glottis secondary to velopharyngeal insufficiency. Her habitual pitch was perceptually judged as low for her age. Loudness was within normal limits.

Copyright © 2007 by Mosby, Inc., an affiliate of Elsevier Inc. All rights reserved.

NOTES

TRIAL THERAPY

SUMMARY

RECOMMENDATIONS

Long-term Treatment Goals

Short-term Treatment Goals

Copyright © 2007 by Mosby, Inc., an affiliate of Elsevier Inc. All rights reserved.

UNSOLVED CASE STUDY 4

MUSCLE TENSION APHONIA OF PSYCHOLOGICAL ETIOLOGY*

See page **18** for overview.

BACKGROUND AND REASONS FOR REFERRAL

Colleen, an 11-year-old female sixth-grade student, was seen for a voice evaluation. She presented with sudden onset of voice loss.

HISTORY

Colleen lost her voice suddenly on December 17th. Prior to that she had had a cold and attributed voice loss to laryngitis associated with the cold. Since then she has been aphonic with reports of occasional voicing episodes occurring at school. She did not express great concern about her voice and has managed at school by using her whispered speech or having friends speak for her when a louder voice is needed. She has not been absent from school or social events. She said that her throat gets dry but does not hurt. Colleen denied any upsetting events or feelings of stress preceding or following the onset of her voice loss. She has had two laryngeal examinations, both with normal findings.

Medical history was negative for reflux, allergies, and asthma. No swallowing problems were reported. No health problems were present, nor have there been recent surgeries or trauma involving the head or neck. Voice abuse was not reported before voice loss.

The client described herself as "accident prone," having experienced numerous orthopedic maladies during the past year. Colleen's mother reported that Colleen is happy and well liked and is a good student. She stated that their home is very busy with two children involved in multiple activities. Additionally, Colleen's mom and dad have been very involved in planning their son's Bar Mitzvah. The mother reported that there is ongoing competition and jealousy between Colleen and her brother.

OBSERVATIONS

The client did not appear upset by her voice, nor did she appear motivated to produce a better voice. She whispered with ease throughout the 60-minute evaluation. Her mother appeared very concerned about Colleen and was observed to sigh repeatedly throughout the appointment, becoming tearful at the end, when improved voice was not achieved.

EVALUATION
Pitch

Unable to determine because of aphonia.

Quality

An effortful whispered quality was audible and consistent throughout the evaluation. No true voice was heard on exhalation. There was one instance of phonation accompanying her attempt to model the clinician's phonation of inhalation. Once she heard her voice, all other attempts to voice on inhalation were unsuccessful. Strong cough and throat clear were heard.

Loudness

Unable to determine because of aphonia.

---

*There is no audio sample because of Colleen's whispered voice.

Copyright © 2007 by Mosby, Inc., an affiliate of Elsevier Inc. All rights reserved.

Respiration

Breathing during rest was appropriate.

Musculoskeletal Tension

Elevated laryngeal position with reduced thyrohyoid space. Exaggerated pain response was noted during laryngeal massage with no voice improvement achieved.

Vocal Abuse Behaviors

Use of effortful whisper.

TRIAL THERAPY

SUMMARY

RECOMMENDATIONS

Long-term Treatment Goals

Short-term Treatment Goals

Copyright © 2007 by Mosby, Inc., an affiliate of Elsevier Inc. All rights reserved.

UNSOLVED CASE STUDY 5

JUVENILE RESONANCE DISORDER

Voice clip #25

OVERVIEW

Juvenile resonance disorder, also known as immature voice, is a disorder unique to postpubescent females. It is sometimes classified and described as a type of puberphonia. The speech characteristics are a higher pitched voice than one would expect for an adult female and a more forward-focused articulation and resonance pattern.[15,17] Typically, excess muscle tension is perceived in the voice and resonance, adding roughness and breathiness to the voice quality. Often nonverbal mannerisms lack maturity as well. The overall impression given by the speaker is that she is much younger than her chronological age. One client receiving therapy stated that when she phoned a hair salon to set up an appointment she was asked if her mommy knew that she was making the appointment!

Therapy by the speech-language pathologist for this disorder should focus on voice, resonance, and articulation. Habitual speaking pitch should be lowered to the pitch that is optimal for the client's vocal folds. Resonance and articulation should be altered by having the speaker open her mouth more when she speaks and establishing a more posterior tongue carriage with firmer articulator contacts. If it appears that there are psychogenic issues associated with the client's voice, a referral to a psychologist or counselor is important.

BACKGROUND AND REASONS FOR REFERRAL

Kasey, a 17-year-old female, was seen for a voice evaluation. The chief complaint was a quiet, high-pitched voice that is negatively impacting her life. Her father accompanied her to this evaluation.

HISTORY

Kasey described her voice as "small" and "squeaky" and said that attempts to talk louder result in a strained feeling. People often ask her to repeat what she has said. Occasionally she yells from one room to another; however, overall she is soft spoken. According to client report, her voice has negatively affected her school experience and her relationship with peers. Her nickname is "Squeak." Her dad reported that teachers throughout her school history have commented on her quiet voice and its impact on school performance.

Kasey stated that she is healthy and has had no trauma or surgeries involving the head or neck. She denied dysphagia, reflux, or allergy symptoms. She is on no medications and denies cigarette and alcohol use. Flexible nasolaryngoscopy revealed her larynx structure and function to be within normal limits for her age and gender. The client stated that a relative also has a "small voice."

Kasey described her personality as quiet, friendly, and ambitious. She attends a performing arts school where she studies drawing. Additionally, she works as a sales associate in a clothing store. She has never had public speaking or singing training, nor has she had speech or voice therapy. She recently expressed an interest in receiving voice therapy to her father.

EVALUATION
Pitch

Speaking fundamental frequency for sustained /a/ was 278 Hz, which is high for same-aged females. Fundamental frequency phonation range was 208-581 Hz. Frequency perturbation was 0.33. A reduction in pitch inflections was heard. Speaking fundamental frequency was reduced when the clinician manually lowered Kasey's larynx position.

Copyright © 2007 by Mosby, Inc., an affiliate of Elsevier Inc. All rights reserved.

Quality

Perceptually, mild breathiness was heard. No hoarseness or voice breaks were noted.

Loudness

Perceptually judged as reduced during conversational speech. Best loudness was heard when Kasey simulated yelling to her mother.

Respiration

Normal abdominothoracic breathing patterns were observed at rest. Maximum sustained /a/ was 8.5 seconds, which is not within normal limits. Sustained /s/ was 18 seconds.

Musculoskeletal Tension

Elevated larynx position, with reduced thyrohyoid space. Discomfort was reported with laryngeal massage.

Vocal Abuse Behaviors

None reported.

Voice Handicap Index

The Voice Handicap Index (VHI) scale, which seeks to assess the level of impact caused by the voice problem within three areas: physical, emotional, and functional, was rated by the client on a 0 to 4 severity level.
Total VHI score: 37/120
> *Subscale scores:*
> 18/40 Emotional
> 12/40 Functional
> 7/40 Physical

Resonation

A forward, high tongue carriage in conjunction with reduced mouth opening and increased nasality of a functional nature contribute to an immature "whining" sound.

Articulation

No articulation errors observed. Significantly decreased movement of her maxilla was noted in all speech contexts, resulting in a "closed" articulation posture.

Hearing Acuity

Pure tone screening of speech frequencies revealed hearing within normal limits bilaterally.

Copyright © 2007 by Mosby, Inc., an affiliate of Elsevier Inc. All rights reserved.

TRIAL THERAPY

SUMMARY

RECOMMENDATIONS

Long-term Treatment Goals

Short-term Treatment Goals

Copyright © 2007 by Mosby, Inc., an affiliate of Elsevier Inc. All rights reserved.

MUSCLE TENSION DYSPHONIA

 Voice clip #26

See page **18** for overview.

BACKGROUND AND REASONS FOR REFERRAL

Pastor Anne, a 35-year-old female, was seen for a voice evaluation upon recommendation from her physician. Anne has had several periods of hoarseness throughout the past year and has expressed an interest in voice care and projection techniques.

HISTORY

According to client report, Pastor Anne has noticed a gradual negative change in voice performance during the past several years. This past year "three bouts of hoarseness" have interfered with her daily vocal demands as a minister. She attributes the problem to voice overuse and vocal strain associated with public speaking. In addition to a hoarse voice quality, after excessive voice use, she clears her throat frequently. Ear, nose, and throat (ENT) examination revealed mild edema and erythema of the vocal cords with no evidence of reflux.

Pastor Anne uses her voice excessively throughout the week with one-on-one, small, and large group gatherings, usually without the aid of an amplification system. When preaching alternate Sundays, she preaches three services, with additional voice use throughout that same day. She frequently has evening meetings throughout the week. She rests her voice on Mondays, the only day of the week that she doesn't work.

The client is in good health. She had her adenoids removed as a teenager. She has had no other hospitalizations. She has no known allergies or symptoms of gastroesophageal reflux. She drinks approximately 6 glasses of water and 3 caffeinated beverages daily. She does not smoke nor is she exposed to second-hand smoke. Vitamins are the only medication taken daily. She enjoys running to relieve stress. She recognizes the stress associated with her profession and is actively working on channeling this appropriately. She has had no formal public speaking or singing training aside from "voice tips" given in seminary.

EVALUATION
Pitch

Speaking fundamental frequency for sustained /a/ was 200 Hz. Habitual pitch for contextual speech was measured at 185 Hz. When speaking at the lower pitch, few downward inflections were heard, and voice sounded less energized. Fundamental frequency pitch range was 150-787 Hz. Frequency perturbation for /a/ was 0.73.

Quality

Perceptually voice quality was within normal limits for conversational speech. Mild roughness was heard on sustained vowels. Speech was articulated in a very deliberate manner causing frequent hard glottal attacks.

Loudness

Mean overall loudness was 81 dB. The client stated that she has a tendency to talk loudly.

Copyright © 2007 by Mosby, Inc., an affiliate of Elsevier Inc. All rights reserved.

Respiration

Appropriate for speech purposes. Maximum phonation duration for /a/ was 12 seconds. S/Z ratio was 0.64 (18 and 28 seconds, respectively).

Vocal Abuse Behaviors

The following abuses were identified and rated on a 0 to 5 scale (5 most frequently occurring).

4—Talking loudly; talking over noise; phone use

Voice Handicap Index

The Voice Handicap Index (VHI) scale, which seeks to assess the level of impact caused by the voice problem within three areas: physical, emotional, and functional, was rated by the client on a 0 to 4 severity scale (0 = never; 4 = always).

Total VHI score: 28/120

Subscale scores:

18/40 Physical

06/40 Functional

04/40 Emotional

Resonation

Within normal limits.

Articulation

Within normal limits.

Copyright © 2007 by Mosby, Inc., an affiliate of Elsevier Inc. All rights reserved.

TRIAL THERAPY

SUMMARY

RECOMMENDATIONS

Long-term Treatment Goals

Short-term Treatment Goals

Copyright © 2007 by Mosby, Inc., an affiliate of Elsevier Inc. All rights reserved.

UNSOLVED CASE STUDY 7

VOCAL POLYP

 Voice clip #27

OVERVIEW

Vocal fold polyps are often similar to nodules with regard to etiology: voice abuse and misuse causing excessive muscle tension. Most polyps develop gradually, though occasionally they follow a single voice abuse episode. Some polyps are sessile, meaning that they have a broad base similar to nodules, originating in the cover of the vocal fold. They often appear on the free edge of the vocal fold at the anterior third, posterior two-thirds junction where the vocal folds vibrate with greatest force. They are most often unilateral and larger than a nodule. Some polyps are pedunculated, which means attached from a stalk. They may be on the free edge of the vocal fold or they also can be elsewhere in the larynx. When on the underside of the vocal fold, they often are only visualized with phonation when the airflow "blows" the polyp to where it is visible. Polyps that appear blood filled are called *hemorrhagic polyps*.

Perceptual voice characteristics caused by a polyp will vary depending on the size and location of the polyp. If on the free edge of the vocal fold, it is anticipated that the voice will sound rough because of the added mass on one fold affecting the periodicity of vibration, and breathy because of the incomplete glottal closure as the folds try to close around the polyp. The added mass will reduce speaking fundamental frequency and affect phonation range. If the polyp is large, it may vibrate and have a mucosal wave independent of the rest of the vocal fold. The speaker will frequently complain of poor voice quality, vocal fatigue, and the need to clear the throat in response to a feeling that something is there.

Often polyps are removed surgically. A course of voice therapy before surgery reduces swelling and irritation of the area surrounding and opposing the polyp and educates the client on postoperative voice care. Voice therapy after surgical removal of the polyp targets the reduction of vocal hyperfunction and the improvement of vocal hygiene.

BACKGROUND AND REASONS FOR REFERRAL

Brittney, a 19-year-old female, was seen for a voice evaluation on recommendation from her otolaryngologist. The presenting complaints were chronic laryngitis and intermittent voice loss. She has been diagnosed with a unilateral sessile polyp.

HISTORY

Brittney initially received voice therapy at this clinic for vocal nodules 5 years before this evaluation. Upon dismissal from therapy, her voice was within normal limits, and her vocal folds were without evidence of nodules. During the past year, the client reports a gradual worsening in voice quality with periods of voice loss. She recently completed her freshman year at a large university. Brittney attributes voice problems to excessive loud talking and yelling at sporting events. She noted these symptoms: throat irritation and dryness and hoarseness and voice loss that is worse in the morning and again late at night. The client describes herself as "very social."

History is negative for cigarette and alcohol use. Caffeine intake is estimated as less than one beverage per day. Noncaffeinated fluid intake is high (six glasses of water per day). Seasonal allergies are not reported, nor does she have overt symptoms of reflux. Prednisone was taken for approximately 2 weeks after the polyp diagnosis to reduce vocal fold swelling. During that time, she noted an improvement in her voice quality; however, it was not long lasting.

Copyright © 2007 by Mosby, Inc., an affiliate of Elsevier Inc. All rights reserved.

Brittney is involved in mentoring youth, where she frequently acts as a group discussion and activity leader. She participated as a camp leader for 1 week earlier this summer where she stated that by midweek she had complete voice loss.

EVALUATION
Pitch

Speaking fundamental frequency for sustained /a/ was 201 Hz. Fundamental frequency pitch range was 157-678 Hz. Frequency perturbation for /a/ was 1.61.

Quality

For sustained vowels, roughness was rated as 2 (mild to moderate), whereas breathiness was rated as 3 (moderate). While reading sentences and a passage, roughness was rated as 3 (moderate) and breathiness as 2 (mild to moderate). Strain was rated as 3 (moderate). Glottal fry was noted at the end of breath groups. Glottal attacks and phonation breaks were heard. Voice quality was consistent throughout the evaluation.

Loudness

Inappropriately loud for a conversational setting. She evidenced a loud, hearty laugh (74-88 dB) frequently throughout the evaluation.

Respiration

Appropriate for speech purposes; /a/ was sustained for 18 seconds; S/Z ratio was 1.3 (29 and 22 seconds, respectively). Functionally, she was observed to talk until expiratory reserve volume appears depleted, resulting in increased effort and glottal fry phonation toward the end of breath groups.

Vocal Abuse Behaviors

The following abuses were identified and rated on a 0 to 5 scale (5 most frequently occurring).

  5—Talking loudly; talking excessively
  4—Shouting/screaming; talking over noise; making noises; using different voices
  3—Throat clearing

Voice Handicap Index

The Voice Handicap Index (VHI) scale, which seeks to assess the level of impact caused by the voice problem within three areas: physical, emotional, and functional, was rated by the client on a 0 to 4 severity scale (0 = never; 4 = always).
Total VHI score: 32/120
  Subscale scores:
  19/40 Physical
  07/40 Functional
  06/40 Emotional

Copyright © 2007 by Mosby, Inc., an affiliate of Elsevier Inc. All rights reserved.

TRIAL THERAPY

SUMMARY

RECOMMENDATIONS

Long-term Treatment Goals

Short-term Treatment Goals

Copyright © 2007 by Mosby, Inc., an affiliate of Elsevier Inc. All rights reserved.

NOTES

UNSOLVED CASE STUDY 8

VOCAL FOLD PARALYSIS

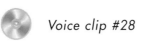 *Voice clip #28*

See page **55** for overview.

BACKGROUND AND REASONS FOR REFERRAL

Evan, a 19-year-old college freshman, was seen for a voice evaluation, stating that he would like a "better voice." He has a diagnosis of a complete left vocal fold adductor paralysis and a near total right vocal fold adductor paralysis.

HISTORY

Evan was born prematurely, with a very low birth weight. He was intubated for approximately 6 weeks and subsequently had a tracheotomy for about 2½ years. It is not known whether vocal cord paralysis was congenital or iatrogenic.

In early childhood, Evan was apparently able to create a "rough voice" by using supraglottic phonation. Through speech therapy, use of the "rough voice" was discouraged, and his true voice, which was a whisper, was encouraged. Subsequently, he discontinued using supraglottic phonation.

Vocal cord medialization surgery was performed 1 year before this evaluation. Two attempts to medialize the left vocal fold were unsuccessful.

Evan's most recent laryngeal examination was performed 2 months before this evaluation at a very reputable voice center. Results of the examination indicated that Evan's right vocal fold is capable of moving from an abducted to a 30% adducted position, and his left vocal fold is completely immobile. During the time of the examination, while his airway was anesthetized, before stroboscopy, Evan was able to produce supraglottic phonation, which was surprisingly loud and functional. Subsequent to that, it was recommended that Evan attempt to discover to what extent supraglottic phonation might be achievable through voice therapy.[61]

Evan does not smoke. Noncaffeinated fluid intake is good. He takes no medications. He reports no swallowing problems but states that he is careful when drinking liquids.

Evan is currently studying information technology. He is enjoying college, where he is a resident student. He has never received counseling for his communication disability.

OBSERVATIONS

The client appeared healthy. He willingly participated in all voice tasks. He was noted to have a residual scar from his tracheotomy. He also had a small scar on the left side of his neck from the thyroplasty procedure.

EVALUATION (NONSUPRAGLOTTIC VOICE)
Pitch

Fundamental frequency for sustained /a/ was 118 Hz. Habitual pitch for contextual speech was measured at 109 Hz. Evan was able to produce his lowest voice at 98 Hz and his highest at 147 Hz, a range of seven notes.

Quality

Evan spoke in an aphonic voice. Breathiness and strain were rated as 5 (severe). Roughness was rated as 2 (mild to moderate). Frequency perturbation was measured at 8.42, which greatly exceeds normal limits and correlates perceptually with extreme breathiness.

Copyright © 2007 by Mosby, Inc., an affiliate of Elsevier Inc. All rights reserved.

Loudness

Quiet for a small group setting. During contextual speech, Evan's habitual loudness was 66.09 dB. His dynamic range (softest to loudest voice) when sustaining /a/ was 64-74 dB, whereas the normal range is 50-115 dB SPL (sound pressure level).

Respiration

Abdominothoracic breathing is observed. Due to lack of laryngeal valving, reduced utterance length per breath was observed when speaking and reading. Maximum phonation duration for /a/ was 3.5 seconds.

Resonation

Within normal limits without hypernasality.

Articulation

Within functional limits; mild articulation distortion heard on /r/ phoneme.

TRIAL THERAPY

Supraglottic phonation was explained and varying facilitative techniques were introduced. Most success was experienced when using an effortful throat clear to achieve phonation. Acoustic data generated from Evan's production of supraglottic phonation is as follows:

Habitual Pitch

81 Hz

Intensity

82 dB

Frequency Perturbation

4.11

Maximum Phonation Duration

5.25 sec

Copyright © 2007 by Mosby, Inc., an affiliate of Elsevier Inc. All rights reserved.

SUMMARY

RECOMMENDATIONS

Long-term Treatment Goals

Short-term Treatment Goals

Copyright © 2007 by Mosby, Inc., an affiliate of Elsevier Inc. All rights reserved.

UNSOLVED CASE STUDY 9

VOCAL NODULES POSTSURGERY

    Voice clip #29

See page **36** for overview.

BACKGROUND AND REASONS FOR REFERRAL

Paul, a 42-year-old instrumental music teacher, singer, and saxophonist, was seen for a voice evaluation. The presenting complaints were hoarseness and a reduced ability to sing, following surgical removal of bilateral vocal fold nodules.

HISTORY

According to client report, vocal nodules were removed 2 months before this evaluation. Voice therapy was not recommended or received before surgery to remove his nodules. At a follow-up appointment with his otolaryngologist, Paul expressed his dissatisfaction regarding his voice, which prompted his physician to suggest voice therapy. According to Paul, his most recent laryngeal examination revealed redness and swelling of both vocal folds. Laryngeal stroboscopy has not been performed.

After surgery, Paul briefly rested his voice but then resumed teaching 5 days per week, playing in clubs 4 evenings per week, and singing with a choir on occasional Sundays. Presently Paul is not singing but continues to play the saxophone. He has made modifications while teaching that include using amplification and vocalizing less. He continues to experience hoarseness and feels discouraged and concerned.

History is negative for alcohol use. Exposure to second-hand smoke is experienced both at home and in clubs. Daily intake of caffeine is 60 ounces of coffee and 24 ounces of soda. No more than one glass of water a day is consumed. The client has a generalized anxiety disorder for which he takes Effexor 75 mg. During the past year his son was diagnosed with juvenile diabetes, which has been upsetting to Paul.

Paul presents with a gregarious personality. He stated, however, that not being able to sing has upset him greatly. He brought a CD of his singing voice before voice problems with him to this evaluation. His vocal range was that of a baritone with a very resonant tone that covered three octaves with ease.

EVALUATION
Pitch

Fundamental frequency for sustained /a/ was 109 Hz. Fundamental frequency pitch range was 85-404 Hz with a break when transitioning from chest to head voice. Singing range, for which he had control, was nine notes. Frequency perturbation for /a/ was 2.46.

Quality

Perceptual rating for hoarseness was moderate to severe (4), whereas breathiness was rated as moderate (3). Frequent phonation breaks were heard.

Loudness

Appropriate for a quiet setting with no background noise. The client stated that when he talks loudly, he feels vocal strain.

Respiration

Abdominothoracic breathing noted. Maximum phonation duration for /a/ was 20 seconds. S/Z ratio was 1.48 (20 and 13.5 seconds, respectively).

Copyright © 2007 by Mosby, Inc., an affiliate of Elsevier Inc. All rights reserved.

Vocal Abuse Behaviors

The following abuses were identified and rated on a 0 to 5 scale (5 most frequently occurring).
> 5—Talking excessively
> 4—Loud talking, talking over noise
> 3—Shouting, yelling, singing

Musculoskeletal Tension

Palpation of the larynx revealed an elevated position with a reduced and hardened thyrohyoid space. Mild pain was expressed during palpation.

Voice Handicap Index

The Voice Handicap Index (VHI) scale, which seeks to assess the level of impact caused by the voice problem within three areas: physical, emotional, and functional, was rated by the client on a 0 to 4 severity scale.

Total VHI score: 77/120
> *Subscale scores:*
> 35/40 Physical
> 26/40 Emotional
> 16/40 Functional

Copyright © 2007 by Mosby, Inc., an affiliate of Elsevier Inc. All rights reserved.

TRIAL THERAPY

SUMMARY

RECOMMENDATIONS

Long-term Treatment Goals

Short-term Treatment Goals

Copyright © 2007 by Mosby, Inc., an affiliate of Elsevier Inc. All rights reserved.

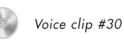

UNSOLVED CASE STUDY 10

PARKINSON DISEASE

Voice clip #30

OVERVIEW

Parkinson disease is a progressive basal ganglia disease caused by a depletion of dopamine (needed for neural transmission) and has a gradual onset of symptoms that affect movement as well as communication. The most common symptoms are slowed movement (bradykinesia), rigidity observed in movement, posture, and facial expression, reduced range of motion, and a resting tremor.

The voice and speech symptoms, classified as *hypokinetic dysarthria*, are sometimes the first signs of disease onset. Voice is often breathy because of a bowed or open glottal chink vocal fold closure pattern resulting from antagonistic rigidity between the adductor and abductor intrinsic laryngeal muscles.[25] There may be vocal roughness as well. A decrease in overall loudness is noted. Fewer pitch and loudness inflections are heard. Rate increases as the speaker continues to talk, with reduced awareness of breath control. A tremor may be present in the voice. Articulation may lack precision and the client may report dysphagia symptoms.

Management of Parkinson disease is accomplished initially through medication, which provides dopamine to the body. Neurosurgical procedures are being offered as well, to provide systemic benefits. If the speaker's voice is extremely breathy and dysphagia is reported, vocal fold augmentation will improve glottal closure.

Voice therapy for Parkinson disease has been reported on extensively, based on the positive efficacy studies conducted on the Lee Silverman Voice Therapy Program[59,60] for Parkinson disease. This program, which requires the clinician to have specific training in its use, emphasizes the development and use of a loud voice, which in so doing improves other negative aspects of the hypokinetic dysarthria.

This author has found vocal function exercises[69] to be helpful in the treatment of the voice of the Parkinson client when used in conjunction with therapy techniques that focus on correct (nonstrained) use of a loud voice; rate and breath control management; and exaggerated articulator movement. Teaching the speaker to "recalibrate" his kinesthetic and auditory feedback systems, to promote carryover into "nontherapy" settings, remains challenging.

BACKGROUND AND REASONS FOR REFERRAL

Harry, a 73-year-old retired educator, was seen for a voice evaluation and cognitive screening secondary to a diagnosis of Parkinson disease. His chief complaint is a "weak" voice.

HISTORY

Approximately 3 years ago, Harry first noticed a tremor in his hands. He also felt that he was "less limber," taking longer to accomplish motor tasks that he had once done with ease. He went to his internist and was told that his symptoms most likely suggested Parkinson disease. Harry has a family history of this. He was referred to a neurologist, who confirmed the diagnosis. He was started on the medication Sinemet. Since that time, his symptoms have progressed. Presently Harry uses a walker and has increased difficulty transferring from one position to another. He also noted that his voice has become very weak, which interferes with communication between his wife and himself. When he attempts to talk loudly, he quickly "runs out of air." His medication has been increased, which reduces the tremor in his extremities and aids his locomotion. He did not report swallowing problems.

Copyright © 2007 by Mosby, Inc., an affiliate of Elsevier Inc. All rights reserved.

Harry is alert, attentive, and motivated to improve his speech. He has had no previous speech therapy. He wears bifocals. His hearing appears to be within functional limits. He attends a senior day center 3 days per week, where he participates in physical and recreational therapy.

EVALUATION
Pitch

Speaking fundamental frequency for sustained /a/ was 130 Hz, and judged perceptually as within normal limits. Phonation range was 110-190 Hz, without pitch or phonation breaks.

Quality

Overall severity was rated as 3 (moderate). Breathiness was rated as 3 (moderate), whereas roughness was rated as 1 (mild). No tremor, voice spasms, or strain were noted.

Loudness

Perceptually judged as quiet and rated as 3 (moderate) for a small group setting without background noise. Moderate asthenia was noted with continued voice use. Loudness was noted to decay, with each breath group starting audibly and regressing to a whisper.

Respiration

Thoracic breathing with increased effort was observed. Mean phonation duration for /a/ was 4 seconds. Mean sustained /s/ was 11 seconds.

Vocal Abuse Behaviors

None reported.

Resonation

Within normal limits without hypernasality.

Articulation

Reduced diadochokinetic rate and precision heard on individual syllables and the multisyllabic target. Reduced force of articulation noted on fricatives. Speech intelligibility was good.

Rate

When conversing, rate was appropriate at the outset of speech but became increasingly rapid with continued speech.

COGNITIVE SCREENING

Portions of the Ross Information Processing Assessment—Geriatric[70] were administered, yielding the following interpretation: Performance was within normal limits for verbal expression, word recall, auditory comprehension, problem solving, word fluency, and orientation. Mild deficits in short-term auditory memory were noted.

Copyright © 2007 by Mosby, Inc., an affiliate of Elsevier Inc. All rights reserved.

TRIAL THERAPY

SUMMARY

RECOMMENDATIONS

Long-term Treatment Goals

Short-term Treatment Goals

Copyright © 2007 by Mosby, Inc., an affiliate of Elsevier Inc. All rights reserved.

UNSOLVED CASE STUDY SCORING RUBRIC

4 = Thorough and accurate (Very good)

3 = Met assignment guidelines (Good)

2 = Touched upon briefly (Satisfactory)

1 = Lacked clarity/erroneous (Poor)

0 = omitted this information

Group or Individual Presenter: _____   **Grade:** _____

Trial Therapy:	4	3	2	1	0
Summary:	4	3	2	1	0
Recommendations:	4	3	2	1	0
Long-term Goal(s):	4	3	2	1	0
Short-term Goal(s):	4	3	2	1	0

Treatment Plan:

Therapy Technique(s): _____

Appropriate to disorder?	yes	no			
Appropriate to the client?	yes	no			
Efficacious?	yes	no			
Hierarchy reflects thought?	4	3	2	1	0
Materials:	4	3	2	1	0
Demonstration:	4	3	2	1	0
Method for documentation:	yes	no			
Bibliography (APA):	4	3	2	1	0
Oral Presentation:	4	3	2	1	0
Handout/PowerPoint:	4	3	2	1	0

Comments:

Copyright © 2007 by Mosby, Inc., an affiliate of Elsevier Inc. All rights reserved.

1. American Speech-Language-Hearing Association: *Evidence-based practice in communication disorders: position statement*, 2005. Retrieved February 27, 2006, from http://www.asha.org/members/deskrefjournals/deskref/default

2. American Speech-Language-Hearing Association: *HIPAA: general information*, n.d. Retrieved February 25, 2006, from http://www.asha.org/about/legislation-advocacy/federal/hipaa/hippa_general_faq.htm

3. American Speech-Language-Hearing Association: Knowledge and skills for speech-language pathologists with respect to evaluation and treatment for tracheoesophageal puncture and prosthesis, *ASHA Supplement* 24:166-177, 2004.

4. American Speech-Language-Hearing Association: *New certification standards*, 2006. Retrieved February 28, 2006, from http://www.asha.org/about/membership-certification/new_standards.htm

5. American Speech-Language-Hearing Association: *Preferred practice patterns for the profession of speech-language pathology*, 2004. Retrieved February 28, 2005, from http://www.asha.org/members/deskref-journal/deskref/default

6. American Speech-Language-Hearing Association: Vocal tract visualization and imaging: position statements, *ASHA Supplement* 24:64, 2004.

7. American Speech-Language-Hearing Association Special Interest Division 3, Voice and Voice Disorders: *Consensus auditory-perceptual evaluation of voice (CAPE-V) form*, 2003. Retrieved February 25, 2006, from http://www.asha.org/NR/rdonlyres/79EE699E-DAEE-4E2C-C11BDE6B1D67/ 0/CAPEV

8. American Speech-Language-Hearing Association Special Interest Division 3, Voice and Voice Disorders: *Consensus auditory-perceptual evaluation of voice (CAPE-V) instructions*, 2003. Retrieved February 25, 2006, from http://www.asha.org/NR/rdonlyres/3FA67246B-4DA2-84D8-BEFCA5D99345/ 0/CAPEV

9. Andrews M: *Manual of voice treatment—pediatrics through geriatrics*, San Diego, 1995, Singular.

10. Andrews M, Summers A: *Voice treatment for children and adolescents*, San Diego, 2002, Singular.

11. Aronson A: *Clinical voice disorders—an interdisciplinary approach*, ed 3, New York, 1990, Thieme.

12. Belafsky P, Postma G, Koufman J: Validity and reliability of the reflux symptom index (RSI), *J Voice* 16(2):274-277, 2002.

13. Blager FB, Gay ML, Wood RP: Voice therapy techniques adapted to treatment of habit cough: a pilot study, *J Commun Disord* 21(5):393-400, 1988.

14. Bless DM: Assessment of laryngeal function. In Ford CN, Bless DM, editors: *Phonosurgery: assessment and surgical management of voice disorders*, New York, 1991, Raven Press.

15. Boone D, McFarlane S, VonBerg S: *The voice and voice therapy*, ed 7, New Jersey, 2005, Prentice-Hall, Inc.

16. Brugman SM, Simons SM: Vocal cord dysfunction—don't mistake it for asthma, *Phys Sportsmed* 26(5):63-74, 1998.

17. Colton R, Casper J: *Understanding voice problems*, ed 3, Baltimore, Md, 2006, Williams & Wilkins.

18. Cornut G, Bouchayer M: *Assessing dysphonia: the role of videostroboscopy, an interactive video textbook* [motion picture], Lincoln Park, NJ, 2004, Kay Elemetrics.

19. Cymbalta: *Symptoms and causes of depression*, 2005. Retrieved April 20, 2005, from http://www.cymbalta.com/depression/understand/causes.jsp?reqNavId=1.3

20. Daniloff R, Schuckers G, Feth L: *The physiology of speech and hearing: an introduction*, Englewood Cliffs, NJ, 1980, Prentice Hall.

Copyright © 2007 by Mosby, Inc., an affiliate of Elsevier Inc. All rights reserved.

21. Eckel FC, Boone DR: The S/Z ratio as an indicator of laryngeal pathology, *J Speech Hear Disord* 46(2):147-149, 1981.

22. Edgar J, Sapienza C, Bidus K, et al: Acoustic measures of symptoms in abductor spasmodic dysphonia, *J Voice* 15(3):362-372, 2001.

23. Erskine RG, Moursund JP, Trautmann RL: *Beyond empathy: a therapy of contact-in-relationship*, New York, 1999, Brunner-Routledge.

24. Fairbanks G: *Voice and articulation drillbook*, ed 2, New York, 1960, Harper and Brothers.

25. Gallena S, Smith P, Zeffiro T, et al: Effects of levodopa on laryngeal muscle activity for voice onset and offset in Parkinson disease, *J Speech Lang Hear Res* 44(6):1284-1299, 2001.

26. Gallena S, Terrell L, Wolfe M: *Characteristics and treatment effectiveness of children with habit cough*, San Diego, 2005 (November), Poster session presented at American Speech Hearing Association Convention.

27. Golding-Kushner K: *Therapy techniques for cleft palate speech and related disorders*, San Diego, 2001, Singular.

28. Goodglass H: *Boston diagnostic aphasia examination*, ed 3, Philadelphia, 2001, Lippincott Williams & Wilkins.

29. Hanson JT, Lambert DR: *Netter's clinical anatomy*, New Jersey, 2005, Icon Learning System.

30. Hedge MN: *A coursebook on scientific and professional writing in speech-language pathology*, San Diego, 1994, Singular.

31. Heuer R, Towne C, Hockstein N, et al: The Towne-Heuer reading passage—a reliable aid to the evaluation of voice, *J Voice* 14(2):236-239, 2000.

32. Hirano M: *Clinical examination of voice*, New York, 1981, Springer-Verlag.

33. Hixon T, Hoit J: Physical examination of the abdominal wall by the speech-language pathologist, *Am J Speech Lang Path* 8(4):335-346, 1999.

34. Hixon T, Hoit J: Physical examination of the diaphragm by the speech language pathologist, *Am J Speech Lang Pathol* 7(4):37-45, 1998.

35. Hoit JD: Influence of body position on breathing and its implications for the evaluation and treatment of speech and voice disorders, *J Voice* 9(4):341-347, 1995.

36. Jacobson B: The voice handicap index (VHI): development and validation, *Am J Speech Lang Pathol* 6:66-70, 1997.

37. Kaplan E, Goodglass H, Weintraub S: *Boston naming test*, Philadelphia, 1983, Lea & Febiger.

38. Kummer AW: *Cleft palate and craniofacial anomalies: effects on speech and resonance*, Canada, 2001, Singular.

39. Lauver P, Harvey DR: *The practical counselor: elements of effective helping*, Pacific Grove, Calif, 1997, Brooks/Cole.

40. Lopez-Ortiz A: *Frequently asked questions about coffee and caffeine*, 1994. Retrieved February 27, 2006, from http://www.a1b2c3.com/drugs/caff01.htm

41. Ludlow C: Management of the spasmodic dysphonias. In Rubin J, Sataloff R, Korovin G, et al, editors: *Diagnosis and treatment of voice disorders*, New York, 1995, Igaku-Shoin.

42. Mathers-Schmidt B: Paradoxical vocal fold motion: a tutorial on a complex disorder and speech-language pathologist's role, *Am J Speech-Lang Pathol* 10:111-125, 2001.

43. Mathieson L: *The voice and its disorders*, ed 6, London, 2001, Whurr.

44. McNeil MM, Prescott TE: *Revised token test*, Austin, Texas, 1978, Pro-Ed.

45. Meyer SM: *Survival guide for the beginning speech-language clinician*, Gaithersburg, Md, 1998, Aspen.

46. Morrison M, Rammage L: The irritable larynx syndrome, *J Voice* 13(3):447-453, 1999.

47. Morrison M, Nichol H, Rammage L: Diagnostic criteria in functional dysphonia, *Laryngoscope* 94(1):1-8, 1986.

48. National Institute of Mental Health: *Anxiety disorders*, 2006. Retrieved February 25, 2006, from http://www.nimh.nih.gov/healthinformation/anxietymenu.cfm

Copyright © 2007 by Mosby, Inc., an affiliate of Elsevier Inc. All rights reserved.

49. National Institute of Mental Health: *Depression*, 2006. Retrieved February 25, 2006, from http://www.nimh.nih.gov/healthinformation/depressionmenu.cfm

50. Netsell R, Boone D: Dysarthria in adults: physiologic approach to rehabilitation, *Arch Phys Med Rehabil* 60(11):502-508, 1979.

51. Nichols WR, editor: *Webster's college dictionary*, ed 2, New York, 1999, Random House.

52. Noble-Sanderson G: *Voice choice: classroom lessons for the prevention and remediation of vocal abuse*, San Antonio, 1995, The Psychological Corporation.

53. Orlikoff RF, Baken RJ: *Clinical speech and voice measurement: laboratory exercise*, San Diego, 1993, Singular.

54. Pannbacker M: Treatment of vocal nodules: options and outcomes, *Am J Speech Lang Pathol* 8:209-217, 1999.

55. Pannbacker M: Voice treatment techniques: a review and recommendations for outcome studies, *Am J Speech Lang Pathol* 7(3):49-64, 1998.

56. Pindzola R: *A voice assessment protocol for children and adults*, Tulsa, 1987, Modern Education Corporation.

57. Poburka B: A new stroboscopy rating form, *J Voice* 13(3):403-413, 1999.

58. Psych Central: *Facts about anxiety disorders*, 1999. Retrieved April 20, 2005, from http://www.psychcentral.com/disorders/anxietyfacts.htm

59. Ramig LO, Bonitati CM, Lemke JH, et al: Voice treatment for patients with Parkinson disease: development of an approach and preliminary efficacy data, *J Med Speech Lang Pathol* 2(3):191-209, 1994.

60. Ramig LO, Verdolini K: Treatment efficacy: voice disorders, *J Speech Lang Hear Res* 41:S101-S116, 1998.

61. Rammage L, Morrison M, Nichol H, et al: *Management of the voice and its disorders*, ed 2, Vancouver, Canada, 2001, Singular.

62. Roth C: A peek at the status of evidence-based practice in voice treatment, *California Speech Hear Assoc Mag* 34(3), 2005.

63. Roy N, Leeper HA: Effects of the manual laryngeal musculoskeletal tension reduction technique as a treatment for functional voice disorders: perceptual and acoustic measures, *J Voice* 7(3):242-249, 1993.

64. Roy N, Weinrich B, Gray SD, et al: Three treatment techniques for teachers with voice disorders: a randomized clinical trial, *J Speech Lang Hear Res* 46(3): 670-688, 2003.

65. Sapienza C, Walton S, Murry T: Adductor spasmodic dysphonia and muscular tension dysphonia: acoustic analysis of sustained phonation and reading, *J Voice* 14(4):502-520, 2000.

66. Schwartz SK: *The source for voice disorders: adolescent and adult*, East Moline, Ill, 2004, LinguiSystems.

67. Sisterhen D: Clinical use of average fundamental frequency, *Adv Speech-Lang Pathol Audiol* 14(29):16, 2004.

68. Stemple J, Glaze L, Gerdeman B: *Clinical voice pathology: theory and management*, San Diego, 1996, Singular.

69. Stemple J, Lee L, D'Amico B, et al: Efficacy of vocal function exercises as a method of improving voice production, *J Voice* 8:271-278, 1994.

70. Tait N, Michel J, Carpenter M: Maximum duration of sustained /s/ and /z/ in children, *J Speech Hear Disord* 45:239-246, 1980.

71. Verdolini K, Devore K, McCoy S, et al: *Guide to vocology*, Denver, 1998, National Center for Voice and Speech.

72. Verdolini K, Druker D, Palmer P, et al: Laryngeal adduction in resonant voice, *J Voice* 12(3):315-327, 1998.

73. Verdolini K, Rosen C, Branski R: *Classification manual for voice disorders–I*, New Jersey, 2006, Lawrence Erlbaum Associates.

74. Wolfe V, Ratusnik D, Smith F, et al: Intonation and fundamental frequency in male-to-female transsexuals, *J Speech Hear Disord* 55:43-50, 1990.

75. Zwitman D, Calcaterra T: The "silent cough" method for vocal hyperfunction, *J Speech Hear Disord* 38(1):119-125, 1979.

Copyright © 2007 by Mosby, Inc., an affiliate of Elsevier Inc. All rights reserved.

ADDITIONAL READINGS

Adler R, Hirsch S, Mordaunt M: *Voice and communication therapy for the transgender/transsexual client*, San Diego, 2006, Plural Publishing.

Altman K, Mirza N, Ruiz C, Sataloff R: Paradoxical vocal fold motion: presentation and treatment options, *J Voice* 14(1):99-103, 2000.

American Speech-Language-Hearing Association (n.d.): *Praxis exam for speech-language pathologist*. Retrieved February 28, 2006, from www.asha.org/students/praxis/overview.htm

American Speech-Language-Hearing Association: *Code of ethics (revised)*, 2003.

Retrieved February 28, 2005, from http://www.asha.org/members/deskref-journal/deskref/default

Baker J: Psychogenic dysphonia: peeling back the layers, *J Voice* 12(4):527-535, 1998.

Banotai A: Feminization of voice and communication: therapy for transgender clients, *Adv Speech-Lang Pathol Audiol* 15(24):22-25, 2005.

Banotai A (n.d.): Therapy for transgender clients, *Feminization of voice and communication* 15(24):22. Retrieved November 9, 2005, from http://speechlanguage-pathology-audiology.advanceweb.com

Belafsky PC, Postma GN, Koufman JA: Laryngopharyngeal reflux symptoms improve before changes in physical findings, *Laryngoscope* 111(6):979-981, 2001.

Case J: *Clinical management of voice disorders*, ed 2, Austin, Tex, 1991, Pro-Ed.

Champley E: The elicitation of vocal responses from preschool children, *Lang, Speech, Hear Serv Schools* 24:146-150, 1993.

Cooper M: *Stop committing voice suicide*, Los Angeles, 1996, Voice & Speech Company of America.

Freeman M, Fawcus M, editors: *Voice disorders and their management*, ed 3, London, 2001, Whurr.

Hooper C: Changing the speech and language of the male to female transsexual client: a case study, *J Kansas Speech Hear Assoc* 25:1-6, 1985.

Jeffers JD, Laufer RS, editors: *Blakiston's pocket medical dictionary*, ed 4, New York, 1979, McGraw-Hill.

Keith R, Darlely F, editors: *Laryngectomee rehabilitation*, Houston, 1979, College-Hill Press.

Lanter E: Basics of standardized testing part III: many ways to evaluate progress, *Adv Speech-Lang Pathol* 15(35):4-5, 2005.

Lee J: *Culture and sexual orientation*, 2002. Retrieved September 21, 2005, from http://www.asha.org/about/publications/leader-online/archives/2002

Lessac A: *The use and training of the human voice*, New York, 1973, Drama Book Specialists.

Pierce J, Watson T: Psychogenic cough in children: a literature review, *Children's Health Care* 27(1):63–76, 1998.

Rosen C, Murry T, Zinn A, et al: Voice handicap index change following treatment of voice disorders, *J Voice* 14(4):619-623, 2000.

Ross-Swain D, Fogle PT: *Ross information processing assessment—geriatric*, Austin, Tex, 1996, Pro-Ed.

Roy N, Gray SD, Ebert M, et al: An evaluation of the effects of two treatments for teachers with voice disorders: a prospective randomized clinical trial, *J Speech Lang Hear Res* 44(2):286-296, 2001.

Salmon S, Mount K: *Alaryngeal speech rehabilitation*, Austin, Tex, 1991, Pro-Ed.

Copyright © 2007 by Mosby, Inc., an affiliate of Elsevier Inc. All rights reserved.

Schwartz SK: *The source for voice disorders: adolescent and adult*, East Moline, Ill, 2004, LinguiSystems.

Verdolini-Marston K, Burke MK, Lessac A, et al: Preliminary study of two methods of treatment for laryngeal nodules, *J Voice* 9(1):74-85, 1995.

Zemlin W: *Speech and hearing science—anatomy and physiology*, ed 3, Englewood Cliffs, NJ, 1988, Prentice Hall.

Copyright © 2007 by Mosby, Inc., an affiliate of Elsevier Inc. All rights reserved.

Asha Code of Ethics

PREAMBLE

The preservation of the highest standards of integrity and ethical principles is vital to the responsible discharge of obligations by speech-language pathologists, audiologists, and speech, language, and hearing scientists. This Code of Ethics sets forth the fundamental principles and rules considered essential to this purpose.

Every individual who is (a) a member of the American Speech-Language-Hearing Association, whether certified or not, (b) a nonmember holding the Certificate of Clinical Competence from the Association, (c) an applicant for membership or certification, or (d) a Clinical Fellow seeking to fulfill standards for certification shall abide by this Code of Ethics.

Any violation of the spirit and purpose of this Code shall be considered unethical. Failure to specify any particular responsibility or practice in this Code of Ethics shall not be construed as denial of the existence of such responsibilities or practices.

The fundamentals of ethical conduct are described by Principles of Ethics and by Rules of Ethics as they relate to the conduct of research and scholarly activities and responsibility to persons served, the public, and speech-language pathologists, audiologists, and speech, language, and hearing scientists.

Principles of Ethics, aspirational and inspirational in nature, form the underlying moral basis for the Code of Ethics. Individuals shall observe these principles as affirmative obligations under all conditions of professional activity.

Rules of Ethics are specific statements of minimally acceptable professional conduct or of prohibitions and are applicable to all individuals.

PRINCIPLE OF ETHICS I

Individuals shall honor their responsibility to hold paramount the welfare of persons they serve professionally or participants in research and scholarly activities and shall treat animals involved in research in a humane manner.

Rules of Ethics

A. Individuals shall provide all services competently.

B. Individuals shall use every resource, including referral when appropriate, to ensure that high-quality service is provided.

C. Individuals shall not discriminate in the delivery of professional services or the conduct of research and scholarly activities on the basis of race or ethnicity, gender, age, religion, national origin, sexual orientation, or disability.

D. Individuals shall not misrepresent the credentials of assistants, technicians, or support personnel and shall inform those they serve professionally of the name and professional credentials of persons providing services.

E. Individuals who hold the Certificates of Clinical Competence shall not delegate tasks that require the unique skills, knowledge, and judgment that are within the scope of their profession to assistants, technicians, support personnel, students, or any nonprofessionals over whom they have supervisory responsibility. An individual may delegate support services to assistants, technicians, support personnel, students, or any other persons only if those services are adequately supervised by an individual who holds the appropriate Certificate of Clinical Competence.

F. Individuals shall fully inform the persons they serve of the nature and possible effects of services rendered and products dispensed, and they shall inform participants in research about the possible effects of their participation in research conducted.

Copyright © 2007 by Mosby, Inc., an affiliate of Elsevier Inc. All rights reserved.

G. Individuals shall evaluate the effectiveness of services rendered and of products dispensed and shall provide services or dispense products only when benefit can reasonably be expected.

H. Individuals shall not guarantee the results of any treatment or procedure, directly or by implication; however, they may make a reasonable statement of prognosis.

I. Individuals shall not provide clinical services solely by correspondence.

J. Individuals may practice by telecommunication (for example, telehealth/e-health), where not prohibited by law.

K. Individuals shall adequately maintain and appropriately secure records of professional services rendered, research and scholarly activities conducted, and products dispensed and shall allow access to these records only when authorized or when required by law.

L. Individuals shall not reveal, without authorization, any professional or personal information about identified persons served professionally or identified participants involved in research and scholarly activities unless required by law to do so, or unless doing so is necessary to protect the welfare of the person or of the community or otherwise required by law.

M. Individuals shall not charge for services not rendered, nor shall they misrepresent services rendered, products dispensed, or research and scholarly activities conducted.

N. Individuals shall use persons in research or as subjects of teaching demonstrations only with their informed consent.

O. Individuals whose professional services are adversely affected by substance abuse or other health-related conditions shall seek professional assistance and, where appropriate, withdraw from the affected areas of practice.

PRINCIPLE OF ETHICS II

Individuals shall honor their responsibility to achieve and maintain the highest level of professional competence.

Rules of Ethics

A. Individuals shall engage in the provision of clinical services only when they hold the appropriate Certificate of Clinical Competence or when they are in the certification process and are supervised by an individual who holds the appropriate Certificate of Clinical Competence.

B. Individuals shall engage in only those aspects of the professions that are within the scope of their competence, considering their level of education, training, and experience.

C. Individuals shall continue their professional development throughout their careers.

D. Individuals shall delegate the provision of clinical services only to: (1) persons who hold the appropriate Certificate of Clinical Competence; (2) persons in the education or certification process who are appropriately supervised by an individual who holds the appropriate Certificate of Clinical Competence; or (3) assistants, technicians, or support personnel who are adequately supervised by an individual who holds the appropriate Certificate of Clinical Competence.

E. Individuals shall not require or permit their professional staff to provide services or conduct research activities that exceed the staff member's competence, level of education, training, and experience.

F. Individuals shall ensure that all equipment used in the provision of services or to conduct research and scholarly activities is in proper working order and is properly calibrated.

PRINCIPLE OF ETHICS III

Individuals shall honor their responsibility to the public by promoting public understanding of the professions, by supporting the development of services designed to fulfill the unmet needs of the public, and by providing accurate information in all

Copyright © 2007 by Mosby, Inc., an affiliate of Elsevier Inc. All rights reserved.

communications involving any aspect of the professions, including dissemination of research findings and scholarly activities.

Rules of Ethics

A. Individuals shall not misrepresent their credentials, competence, education, training, experience, or scholarly or research contributions.

B. Individuals shall not participate in professional activities that constitute a conflict of interest.

C. Individuals shall refer those served professionally solely on the basis of the interest of those being referred and not on any personal financial interest.

D. Individuals shall not misrepresent diagnostic information, research, services rendered, or products dispensed; neither shall they engage in any scheme to defraud in connection with obtaining payment or reimbursement for such services or products.

E. Individuals' statements to the public shall provide accurate information about the nature and management of communication disorders, about the professions, about professional services, and about research and scholarly activities.

F. Individuals' statements to the public—advertising, announcing, and marketing their professional services, reporting research results, and promoting products—shall adhere to prevailing professional standards and shall not contain misrepresentations.

PRINCIPLE OF ETHICS IV

Individuals shall honor their responsibilities to the professions and their relationships with colleagues, students, and members of allied professions. Individuals shall uphold the dignity and autonomy of the professions, maintain harmonious interprofessional and intraprofessional relationships, and accept the professions' self-imposed standards.

Rules of Ethics

A. Individuals shall prohibit anyone under their supervision from engaging in any practice that violates the Code of Ethics.

B. Individuals shall not engage in dishonesty, fraud, deceit, misrepresentation, sexual harassment, or any other form of conduct that adversely reflects on the professions or on the individual's fitness to serve persons professionally.

C. Individuals shall not engage in sexual activities with clients or students over whom they exercise professional authority.

D. Individuals shall assign credit only to those who have contributed to a publication, presentation, or product. Credit shall be assigned in proportion to the contribution and only with the contributor's consent.

E. Individuals shall reference the source when using other persons' ideas, research, presentations, or products in written, oral, or any other media presentation or summary.

F. Individuals' statements to colleagues about professional services, research results, and products shall adhere to prevailing professional standards and shall contain no misrepresentations.

G. Individuals shall not provide professional services without exercising independent professional judgment, regardless of referral source or prescription.

H. Individuals shall not discriminate in their relationships with colleagues, students, and members of allied professions on the basis of race or ethnicity, gender, age, religion, national origin, sexual orientation, or disability.

I. Individuals who have reason to believe that the Code of Ethics has been violated shall inform the Board of Ethics.

J. Individuals shall comply fully with the policies of the Board of Ethics in its consideration and adjudication of complaints of violations of the Code of Ethics.

From American Speech-Language-Hearing Association: Code of ethics (revised), *ASHA Supplement* 23, pp. 13-15.

Copyright © 2007 by Mosby, Inc., an affiliate of Elsevier Inc. All rights reserved.

Acoustic voice measures—objective assessment of various aspects of voice such as frequency, intensity, and wave complexity

Aerodynamic measures—objective assessment of airflow and air pressure during phonation

Airflow measures—(also known as *aerodynamic measures*) an objective measure that indicates the volume of air moving through the glottis during phonation for a set period, measured in cc or mL per second; high flow volumes and rate are correlated with reduced glottal valving and breathy voice quality, whereas low flow rates are correlated with excessive glottal valving and strained voice quality

Air insufflation test—a diagnostic procedure to assess the muscle tone of the PE segment for alaryngeal speech, whereby air is delivered to the esophagus via a catheter and vibrated at the PE segment

Aphonia—general term indicating an absence of true voice (whisper)

Apnea—cessation of breathing

Botox—a medical treatment used for spasmodic dysphonia that, when injected in minute quantities into the targeted muscle(s), causes a temporary weakness or paralysis of those muscles; also known as *botulinum toxin.*

Brash—the regurgitation of refluxed material into the oral cavity

Consensus auditory perceptual evaluation of voice (CAPE–V)—a perceptual voice assessment tool that allows for severity ratings for minimally five areas of voice and also tallies an overall severity rating

Contact ulcer—unilateral or bilateral ulcerated (depressed) lesion occurring on the cartilaginous portion of the vocal folds at the vocal process of the arytenoids, caused by laryngopharyngeal reflux, intubation trauma, or less commonly by MTD

Cyst (subepithelial)—a benign lesion, usually unilateral, located in the superficial layer of the lamina propria of the vocal fold at the midmembranous junction, causing a rough, breathy voice; it may be misdiagnosed as vocal nodules, especially when there is fullness on the contralateral vocal fold opposing the cyst

Diadochokinesis—rapid repetition of sounds requiring motor agility for successful performance; *speech diadochokinesis:* repetition of pu, tu, ku; *voice diadochokinesis:* repetition of successive /a/ or /i/

Diplophonia—the presence of two pitches produced simultaneously by each vocal fold vibrating at a different frequency

Dynamic range—the range of loudness one's voice can achieve, typically encompassing about 65 dB

Dysphonia—general term for a voice disorder, indicating nonoptimal vocal fold vibration

Dyspnea—difficulty breathing

Edema—swelling

Electrolarynx—a battery-driven instrument that supplies a tone, when the tone generator is placed on the neck, cheek, or inside the mouth; also referred to as *artificial larynx*

Copyright © 2007 by Mosby, Inc., an affiliate of Elsevier Inc. All rights reserved.

Electromyography (EMG)—a procedure conducted by a neurologist using electrodes placed in varying muscles to evaluate the electrical activity of the muscles

Endoscopy—examination of the larynx, pharynx, and nasal area with an endoscope that can be flexible or rigid

Erythema—reddening

Esophageal speech—an alaryngeal method of speech whereby the air, once injected, is held in the upper esophagus and vibrated by the upper esophageal sphincter (PE segment)

Facilitative techniques—voice therapy techniques taught for the express purpose of changing and optimizing vocal fold and laryngeal physiology, thereby achieving a better voice

Falsetto register—the voice register that is higher than the register used for speaking fundamental frequency (chest register)

FVC (forced vital capacity)—a spirometry measurement of the amount of air that one exhales after taking a deep breath; results are based on norms for body size, age, and sex

FEV$_1$ (forced expiratory volume)—a spirometry measurement of the amount of air exhaled in 1 second, which is used in conjunction with FVC to assess airway disease

Fistula—an unintentional or intentional (TE puncture fistula) passage or communication between two parts of the body, or a passage from an internal part to the surface of the body

Flow-volume loop—a method of visually comparing air volume to airflow for forced inhalation and exhalation; a flattened appearance (truncation) of the inspiratory loop signals VCD

Frequency perturbation—(jitter) variability in successive pitch cycles; when outside of normal limits, perturbation is perceived as hoarseness

Functional conversion aphonia—sudden loss of voice despite normal laryngeal structure and function, which has a psychogenic etiology; also known as *muscle tension aphonia* of physiological etiology

Fundamental frequency phonation range—the range of pitches that one's voice is capable of achieving, measured in Hz, determined through the tasks of singing a scale or imitating a siren

Gastroesophageal reflux disease (GERD)—backflow of acidic gastric contents into the esophagus and aerodigestive tract

Globus—a laryngeal sensation of "fullness" or a lump in one's throat, usually associated with laryngopharyngeal reflux

Granuloma(s)—unilateral or bilateral space-occupying lesion occurring at the cartilaginous portion of the vocal folds at the vocal process of the arytenoids caused by laryngopharyngeal reflux (LPR), intubation trauma, or less commonly by MTD

Habit cough—(also referred to as *chronic cough* and *psychogenic cough*) excessive coughing (usually triggered initially by URI) that is absent during sleep, does not respond to medication, but does respond to behavioral therapy

Harmonic:noise ratio—(also known as *signal:noise ratio*) a quantifiable measure of dysphonia in which the harmonics are compared with the noise (roughness, breathiness) of the voice signal

Copyright © 2007 by Mosby, Inc., an affiliate of Elsevier Inc. All rights reserved.

Health Insurance Portability and Privacy Accountability Act (HIPAA)—a federal act that assures privacy practices in health care settings

Hyperfunctional—excessive muscle tension in the absence of pathology

Hypofunctional—inadequate muscle tension in the absence of pathology

Iatrogenic—the etiology (cause) of a problem is the result of a physician's action or medical treatment (example: vocal fold paralysis caused by thyroid surgery)

Idiopathic—the etiology (cause) of the problem is unknown

Intubation—placement of a breathing tube into the trachea for oxygen delivery during surgery or for life support

Irritable larynx syndrome—a laryngeal condition whereby a triggering stimulus causes the larynx and vocal folds to respond with symptoms consistent with vocal cord dysfunction, chronic cough, globus, and MTD

Juvenile resonance disorder—(also known as *immature voice*) a voice resembling that of a child in a postpubescent female, characterized by voice, resonance, and articulation features, that has no organic basis

Klunk—noise made when air enters and opens the PE segment; signals that air has been injected into the upper esophagus

Laryngopharyngeal reflux (LPR)—backflow of stomach acid into the larynx and pharynx causing globus, dysphonia, vocal fatigue

Laryngoscopy—examination of the larynx; **mirror laryngoscopy** requires a small mirror; **flexible laryngoscopy** requires a flexible scope, usually with transnasal placement; **rigid laryngoscopy** uses a rigid straight scope with oral placement

Latency—period of time between air entering the esophagus and voice being heard

Maximum phonation duration (MPD)—length of time in seconds that a vowel can be maximally sustained; influenced by glottal closure pattern and respiratory condition, as well as age and gender

Muscle tension dysphonia (MTD)—voice disorder caused by hyperfunction of the vocal folds and related muscles causing vocal roughness and strain, which may result in structural vocal fold change

Nasal emission—a nasally emitted "air" sound accompanying varying high pressure phonemes, heard in speakers with reduced velopharyngeal competence or occasionally used as a phoneme substitution in a speaker with normal velopharyngeal competence

Neurogenic—of neurological origin

Optimal pitch—the speaking fundamental frequency that requires less effort and results in a "full" sound; unable to be determined in the presence of vocal fold pathology

Organic voice disorder—dysphonia secondary to a structural or systemic disorder or disease

Parkinson disease—a progressive neurological disease caused by reduced levels of dopamine (a neurotransmitter), which results in motor impairments that affect movement and speech

Copyright © 2007 by Mosby, Inc., an affiliate of Elsevier Inc. All rights reserved.

Perceptual voice assessment—subjective description and rating of voice based on the evaluator's trained ear

Pharyngeal flap repair—a surgical procedure used to improve velopharyngeal closure and reduce hypernasal resonance

Pharyngoesophageal segment—(also known as *PE segment; cricopharyngeus* or *upper esophageal sphincter*) the muscle band that connects the pharynx and the esophagus that is the vibratory source for esophageal and TE puncture speech

Phonation breaks—(voice stoppages) episodes of aphonia ranging in duration from a sound to several words; most often associated with excessive laryngeal tension

Phonosurgery—surgery performed on the vocal folds using instruments and techniques designed to promote optimal vocal fold healing, vibration, and closure

Physiological measures—assessment of laryngeal function and vocal fold vibratory characteristics

Pitch break—sudden unpredictable change in pitch that occurs while speaking or singing

Polyp(s)—a unilateral or bilateral, sessile or pedunculated space-occupying lesion occurring in the superficial layer of the lamina propria, secondary to vocal abuse and misuse

Polypoid degeneration—(also called *Reinke's edema*) a swelling of the membranous portion of the vocal folds in Reinke's space caused by the combined effect of improper voice use and chemical irritants (smoking and alcohol use)

Psychogenic—of psychological origin

Puberphonia—maintenance of an inappropriately high-pitched voice after laryngeal growth that accompanies puberty; also referred to as *mutational falsetto* or *functional falsetto*

Pulmonologist—a medical doctor who specializes in diseases of the respiratory system

Radical neck dissection—a surgical procedure to remove malignant lymph nodes from the neck

Recurrent respiratory papilloma (RRP)—viral, wartlike benign growths occurring in the airway that require aggressive management and often recur; when on the vocal folds, voice is dysphonic or aphonic

Reflux Symptom Index—a self-rated measure of reflux symptom severity

S/Z ratio—a comparison of sustained respiration to sustained phonation that provides input regarding the physiology of vocal fold vibration

Shimmer—(also known as *amplitude perturbation*) the cycle-to-cycle variability in the amplitude of vocal fold vibration during sustained vibration; large amounts of shimmer perceptually correlate with dysphonia

Somatoform disorder—a psychogenic displacement (of which the person is unaware) of emotional conflict into physical symptoms, despite normal structure, that is, *conversion voice disorder*

Spasmodic dysphonia—a voice disorder characterized by involuntary adductor and/or abductor spasms of the vocal folds during speech, which has a neurogenic etiology

Copyright © 2007 by Mosby, Inc., an affiliate of Elsevier Inc. All rights reserved.

Speaking fundamental frequency—(also know as *habitual pitch, modal pitch*, or *mean fundamental frequency*) measured in Hz; the average of frequencies used by the speaker in conversational speech

Stoma—an opening in the neck that allows direct access to the trachea for breathing

Strap muscles—extrinsic laryngeal and other muscles of the upper torso that encircle and stabilize the larynx; often a site of tension contributing to MTD

Stridor—noise accompanying inhalation or exhalation that is indicative of upper airway narrowing; often described as wheezing, but different from wheezing

Stroboscopy—a method of visualizing vocal fold vibration through the use of a stroboscope

Supraglottic phonation—vibration of structures above the true vocal folds, which can be symptomatic of MTD, or compensatory for inadequate glottal closure

TNM cancer staging system—a method of staging and reporting the severity of cancer wherein *T* denotes primary tumor site and size, *N* denotes involvement of lymph nodes, and *M* denotes the presence of distant metastasis (spread to other parts of the body)

Temporomandibular joint dysfunction (TMJ)—malfunctioning of the joint wherein the temporal bone meets the mandible, resulting in musculoskeletal tension and pain

Thyrohyoid space—the area between the hyoid bone and thyroid cartilage that is influenced by excessive tension in the laryngeal area

Thyroplasty—a surgical technique to medialize the paralyzed vocal fold toward the midline, thereby improving glottal closure

Total laryngectomy—removal of the entire larynx, including the vocal folds, rendering the person unable to speak by laryngeal means or breathe through the nose or mouth

Tracheoesophageal (TE) puncture—a surgical voice restoration procedure following laryngectomy, wherein a puncture from the trachea to the esophagus allows pulmonary air to travel to the esophagus and be vibrated at the PE segment

Tracheotomy—a procedure whereby a direct opening into the trachea is created, below the vocal folds, for air exchange

Transgendered—a person whose psychological identity is in conflict with biological (anatomical) orientation; MtF means male desiring to be female, whereas FtM denotes female desiring to be male

Tremor—an involuntary, neurologically caused fluctuation in frequency and/or amplitude of vocal fold vibration that can be rhythmic or arrhythmic and differs from vibrato and perturbation

Upper respiratory infection (URI)—a viral or bacterial infection that manifests in cold-type symptoms

Vegetative laryngeal functions—natural sounds produced by the vocal folds, unassociated with speech or singing (laugh, throat clear, cough, grunt, etc.)

Velopharyngeal insufficiency (VPI)—inadequate velopharyngeal valving caused by varying etiologies resulting in hypernasal resonance

Copyright © 2007 by Mosby, Inc., an affiliate of Elsevier Inc. All rights reserved.

Velopharyngeal (VP) prostheses—various types of prostheses (*example:* palatal lift, palatal plates, speech bulbs) worn for purposes of improving VP adequacy and reducing hypernasal resonance

Ventricular phonation—phonation caused by vibration of the ventricular folds; which can be symptomatic of MTD or compensatory for inadequate glottal closure

Vocal cord stripping—a less desirable surgical method used to excise a lesion, affecting the cover of the vocal folds, sometimes resulting in the development of a web or scar tissue

Vocal cord dysfunction (VCD)—(also called *paradoxical vocal fold motion*) a laryngeal disorder whereby the vocal folds adduct on inspiration, causing upper airway compromise and dyspnea; it may accompany strenuous exercise and is frequently misdiagnosed as asthma

Vocal fold augmentation—injecting a substance such as collagen into the paralyzed vocal fold to increase its mass and move it medially, thereby improving glottal closure

Vocal fold paralysis—a neurologically caused motion impairment disorder affecting one or both vocal folds

Vocal nodules—space-occupying lesions, usually bilateral, occurring at the midmembranous junction in the superficial layer of the lamina propria, caused by voice abuse and misuse, resulting in a rough, breathy voice

Voice Handicap Index—a self-rated measure of voice symptom severity consisting of 30 questions divided into functional, physical, and emotional categories that reveals the client's perceived degree of handicap caused by the voice disorder

Copyright © 2007 by Mosby, Inc., an affiliate of Elsevier Inc. All rights reserved.

Page numbers followed by f indicate figures.

Copyright © 2007 by Mosby, Inc., an affiliate of Elsevier Inc. All rights reserved.

Copyright © 2007 by Mosby, Inc., an affiliate of Elsevier Inc. All rights reserved.

Copyright © 2007 by Mosby, Inc., an affiliate of Elsevier Inc. All rights reserved.

Copyright © 2007 by Mosby, Inc., an affiliate of Elsevier Inc. All rights reserved.

Copyright © 2007 by Mosby, Inc., an affiliate of Elsevier Inc. All rights reserved.

Copyright © 2007 by Mosby, Inc., an affiliate of Elsevier Inc. All rights reserved.

Copyright © 2007 by Mosby, Inc., an affiliate of Elsevier Inc. All rights reserved.

CD-ROM Contents

EVALUATION MATERIALS

Adult Case History
Child Case History
Voice Evaluation Form
Stroboscopy Evaluation Rating Form (SERF)
University of Wisconsin Videostroboscopic Ratings
Current Voice Research—ASHA Division 3—CAPE-V
Voice Rating Scale
Rainbow Passage
Towne-Heuer Passage
Voice Handicap Index
Reflux Symptom Index
Speech and Voice Tasks for Assessing Spasmodic Dysphonia
Speech and Voice Tasks for Assessing Resonance
Male-to-Female Transgender Communication Assessment Form
Vocal Cord Dysfunction Patient Interview
Habit Cough Patient Interview

THERAPY MATERIALS

Voice Therapy Progress Note
Treatment for Vocal Cord Dysfunction
Treatment for Habit Cough
Cough Management Chart
Voice Care Tips
Laryngopharyngeal Reflux Information
Sources of Caffeine

LEARNING OPPORTUNITIES (WITH ANSWERS)

Respiration Lab
Voice Analysis Lab
Resonation Lab
Alaryngeal Speech Lab

UNSOLVED CASE STUDIES (WITH ANSWERS)

Unsolved Pediatric Case Studies
Unsolved Adult Case Studies
Unsolved Case Study Scoring Rubric

Copyright © 2007 by Mosby, Inc., an affiliate of Elsevier Inc. All rights reserved.